Conditions, Interpretations and Implications of Normal, Abnormal Determinate and Abnormal Indeterminate Wet Microscopic Urinalysis Findings

Clinical Conditions	Normal	Abnormal Determinate	Abnormal Indeterminate	Clinical Implications
Erythrocyturia	0–3 (Isomorphic)/HPF			Normal
Microhematuria		Dysmorphic RBCs Isomorphic RBCs		Glomerular bleeding Lower urinary tract bleeding
Hematuria		Isomorphic Erythrocytes and Blood Casts Isomorphic Erythrocytes and RTCs		Glomerulopathy; Tubular injury/damage Tubular injury/damage
Gross Hematuria		Explained Hematuria	Unexplained hematuria	Hemorrhage Hemorrhage; Neoplasm
Leukocyturia	0–5 WBCs/HPF			Inflammation; Chronic vs acute inflammation; Inflammatory lesion
		Increased Leukocytes		Inflammation; Inflammatory lesion
Bacteriuria and Leukocyturia		Bacterial UTI		Treatable bacterial UTI
Funguria and Leukocyturia		Fungal UTI		Treatable fungal UTI
Renalcyturia	0–1 Renal cells/HPF	RTCs		Normal Suspect renal injury/damage
Fragments		Benign Urothelial Fragments	Suspect Renal Suspect Abnormal Urothelium	Instrumentation Suspect renal injury/damage Suspect neoplasm
Epithelial Abnormalities			Hypercellularity Abnormal single cells	Neoplasm Neoplasm
Cylinduria (Casts)	0–2 Hyaline/LPF	Increased Hyaline		Normal Dehydration, Congestive heart failure; Stress, Strenuous exercise
	0–2 Granular/LPF	Increased Granular		Normal Dehydration; Stress; Strenuous Exercise
		Heme-granular (Blood)		Renal damage; Glomerulopathy
		Waxy		Chronic renal failure
		Broad		Chronic renal failure
		Cellular (WBCs or RTCs)		Tubulointerstitial inflammation or Tubular injury/damage
		WBCs		Tubulointerstitial inflammation
		Fatty		Nephrotic syndrome
Physiologic Crystalluria		Calcium Oxalate/Monohydrate		Metabolic disorder and/or possible stone former
		Uric Acid		Metabolic disorder and/or possible stone former
		Triple Phosphate		Metabolic disorder and/or possible stone former
Pathologic Crystalluria		Cystine		Cystinuria
		Lysine		Liver disorder
		Tyrosine		Liver disorder
		Cholesterol		Metabolic disorder
Urinary Secretions		Corpora Amylace		Benign prostatic hypertrophy
		Globules		Obstructive uropathy
Lipiduria		Oval Fat Bodies		Nephrotic syndrome
Urinary Concretions		Concretions		Microurolithiasis

Wet Urinalysis

Interpretations, Correlations and Implications

Publishing Team

Erik Tanck (production, illustration, cover)
Terri Horning (production)
Christy Prahl (editorial, proofreading)
Joshua Weikersheimer (consulting publisher)

Notice

Trade names and equipment and supplies described herein are included as suggestions only. In no way does their inclusion constitute an endorsement or preference by the American Society for Clinical Pathology. The ASCP did not test the equipment, supplies, or procedures and, therefore, urges all readers to read and follow all manufacturers' instructions and package insert warnings concerning the proper and safe use of products.

Printed in Hong Kong.

06 05 04 03 5 4 3 2 1

Wet Urinalysis

Interpretations, Correlations and Implications

G Berry Schumann, MD
President and Medical Director
Schumann Diagnostics, Inc
Trumbull, Connecticut

Adjunct Professor
University of Connecticut
School of Allied Health
Storrs, Connecticut

and

Sheryl K Friedman, BS, MT(ASCP)
Technical/Education Coordinator
Dianon Systems, Inc
Stratford, Connecticut

PRESS

American Society for Clinical Pathology
Chicago

Contents

List of Tables

Preface

This compressed but complete handbook was jointly prepared by a senior pathologist/medical scientist and a senior medical technologist/clinical laboratory educator who have a unique experience with frontline wet urinalysis and specialized cytodiagnostic urinalysis. It compiles the most recent physical, chemical and microscopic observations and information regarding wet urinalysis. It also attempts to provide the quickest possible reference to basic differentials and correlations of disorder and findings by putting the inside of the front and rear covers to use! Little space is wasted....

The first chapters ground the reader in the basis of urinalysis, considering signs and symptoms, types of urinalysis, clinical utility, chain of events in urinalysis testing, collection, preservation and transportation of the urine specimen, limitations of the techniques, and a new coordinated approach for wet and cytodiagnostic urinalysis. In addition, a brief review of gross anatomy and histology of the urinary system and a discussion of urine formation is provided.

The middle chapters describe the techniques and their use in greater specific detail. Principles, specificity, and sensitivity of dipstick urinalysis are discussed, with special attention paid to the clinical significance and implications of dipstick urinalysis results and confirmatory chemical testing. The clinical importance of the urine sediment examination and techniques for improved wet urinoscopy are carefully considered. Emphasis is always placed on correlative interpretation of urinary sediment findings, and their implications-including special highlighting of findings that require specific physician or nursing action.

Common urine sediment entities are discussed and illustrated in Chapter 6. A discussion of hematopoietic and epithelial cells, casts, crystals, microorganisms, concretions, and secretions provides quick reference, though the reader is encouraged to consider the larger number of images provided in the differential atlas that is Appendix 2.

Three following chapters present a unique guide for the clinical laboratory practitioner regarding "normal," "abnormal," and "indeterminate" wet urinalysis findings. Correlations of common conditions, urinary system disorders and abnormal wet urinalysis are discussed. But the reader is encouraged to use the correlative tables conveniently provided on the inside of the front cover (for the quickest possible reference!). Chapter 10 concludes the handbook proper with a consideration of quality control and assurance guidelines for wet urinalysis.

The book ends with a glossary and 2 practical appendices. Appendix 1 presents laboratory algorithms for the interpretation and implications of common findings in wet microscopic urinalysis (correlative case reports illustrate the clinical and diagnostic implications of wet urinalysis results). Appendix 2 provides a comparative image atlas to assist the urinoscopist with urine sediment interpretations.

As experienced clinical laboratory professionals involved in specialized cytodiagnostic urinalysis testing, clinical research and education, we strongly believe that when frontline wet urinalysis is properly performed, it will remain the most valuable test in medicine. We hope this book will broaden the diagnostic skills of the urinoscopist and provide new and valuable insights into one of the oldest, and most frequently performed, of all clinical laboratory tests.

Acknowledgments

A pleasant task in completing this new urine pathology handbook is the opportunity to than the numerous contributors whose efforts made this information possible. Although only a few names can be mentioned in print, our grateful appreciation is extended to all involved.

Initially I (GBS) thank John B Henry, MD for supporting my academic career in pathology and laboratory medicine from the very beginning. In addition I thank Leopold G Koss, MD for introducing me to the world of diagnostic cytology and his standard of excellence therein.

I (SKF) thank Mary Bradley, MD for her encouragement in having me learn the importance of urinalysis. Her educational leadership has been a valuable model in my education and training activities. I thank my mentor and coauthor (GBS) for enriching my diagnostic skills by introducing me to a cytologic approach for examining urine sediment.

We would like to pay tribute to Susan C Schweitzer, PhD for her knowledge and guidance regarding renal physiology, urine chemistry, urinalysis quality control and assurance. Her passion and leadership in education and training laboratory professionals on this often neglected laboratory test is valued.

We also gratefully acknowledge the Diagnostic Urocytopathology Laboratory at Dianon Systems (Stratford CT) for access to a wealth of urine samples and experienced laboratory professionals who have dedicated their professional services in defining urine abnormalities and the correlation of frontline wet urinalysis with confirmatory cytodiagnostic urinalysis.

We deeply admire and respect Patricia Merchant who graciously accepted the difficult task of typing the original manuscript.

Most importantly, we are grateful to Joshua Weikersheimer, Publisher for the ASCP Press, for his patience and understanding, and aid in making this book a reality.

Frontline Diagnostic Wet Urinalysis

Urinalysis is the oldest (practiced for some 6000 years) of all medical laboratory tests [Horowitz 1997, Haber 1988]. Although often neglected by clinicians and poorly performed by laboratories, it remains an important, cost-effective, frontline laboratory urine test for screening and initial clinical workup of a variety of renal and lower urinary tract disorders. In terms of the number of tests performed, it remains one of three major in vitro diagnostic screening tests, after serum chemistry profiles and complete blood counts [Kunin 1974]. Recent marketing surveys have estimated that 200 to 300 million urinalyses are performed yearly in the United States [Horowitz 1997]. Ease of specimen collection, low test cost, and rapid turnaround time of test results have contributed to its constant popularity in the initial clinical workup of patients. **T**1.1 provides a comprehensive list of clinical signs and symptoms indicating wet urinalysis. Because urinalysis is fairly simple to perform, easy for the patient, and a noninvasive procedure, it remains a part of the cost-effective approach to clinical medicine.

Laboratory improvements are needed for wet urinalysis to regain its prominence in clinical medicine. Lack of education and training, poorly controlled laboratory methods, and lack of clinically proven diagnostic instrumentation have reduced the value of urinalysis at a time when renal and lower urinary tract diseases are increasing. Accurate and reliable urinalysis testing for the evaluation of kidney disease, bladder cancer, and urinary tract infections is needed, due to the increasing age of our population,

discovery of new clinical disorders, and expanding therapeutic options. Urinalysis must be incorporated into a tangible healthcare plan to provide for the best patient care.

Renal (Kidney) Failure

According to the National Kidney Foundation, at least 20 million Americans suffer from kidney and/or urinary tract related diseases [Schumann 1995]. Thousands of renal transplants are performed for end-stage renal disease each year in the United States alone. Due to the lack of renal transplant donors, there is a growing need for chronic dialysis for end-stage renal disease. While increased awareness and support for renal transplant donors is admirable, and there is hope that "portable," inexpensive dialysis can improve patient lifestyle, the only real solution to renal disease is to prevent it through early detection, and to provide treatment to reverse the disease and delay acute renal failure from progressing to chronic end-stage renal failure. All of these patients can benefit from accurate wet urinalysis testing.

Urinary Tract Infections

Urinary tract infections (UTIs) bring an estimated 6 million patients to physicians' offices annually [Schumann 1995]. The annual cost of lost work hours and wages is staggering. The etiologic agents encountered in the microscopic examination of urine sediment include bacteria, fungi, viruses, and parasites. UTI's are

T1.1 Signs and Symptoms Indicating Wet Urinalysis as a Part of the Diagnostic Workup*

Abdominal pain, acute	Insomnia	Pneumonia
Abdominal pain, chronic recurrent	Jaundice	Polyuria
Abdominal swelling, fecal	Jaw swelling	Precocious puberty
Abdominal swelling, generalized	Joint pain or swelling	Urethral discharge
Absent of diminished pulse	Knee pain	Priapism
Amnesia	Knee swelling	Pruritus, generalized
Anuria or oliguria	Kyphosis	Ptosis
Ascites	Leg Ulceration	Purpura and abnormal bleeding
Back pain	Lip pain	Rales
Bone mass or swelling	Lip swelling	Raynaud's phenomena
Chills	Melena	Rectal discharge
Difficulty urinating	Memory loss	Rectal mass
Dyspareunia	Menorrhagia	Rectal pain
Dysuria (burning or painful)	Meteorism	Respiration abnormalities
Edema, generalized	Metrorrhagia	Restless leg syndrome
Enuresis	Mouth pigmentation	Risus sardonicus
Failure to thrive	Muscular atrophy	Scoliosis
Fever, acute	Musculoskeletal pain, general	Scrotal swelling
Fever, chronic	Nausea, vomiting	Sensory loss
Flank mass	Neck pain	Shoulder pain
Flank pain	Neck swelling	Steatorrhea
Foot ulceration	Nocturia	Stupor
Frequency of urination	Nose, regurgitation of food through	Syncope
Hematuria	Obesity, pathologic	Tachycardia
Hyperpigmentation	Odor	Taste abnormaliites
Hypertension	Opisthotomons	Testicular swelling
Hypotension, chronic	Pain in the penis	Thirst
Hypothermia	Paresthesias of the lower extremity	Thyroid enlargement
Impotence	Paresthesias of the upper extremity	Tongue mass or swelling
Incontinence of urine	Pathologic reflexes	Urethral discharge
Indigestion	Pelvic mass	Urine color changes
Infertility, female	Pelvic pain	Vaginal discharge
Infertility, male	Periorbital edema	Weight loss

*Collins RD. *Algorithmic Diagnosis of Symptoms and Signs: Cost-Effective Approach.* New York: Igaku-Shoin,1995.

routinely encountered in various clinical settings as a primary or concomitant factor associated with complex urinary system disease processes. Terms used to describe the location of UTIs include ureteritis, cystitis, and pyelonephritis (the last, if not corrected, may cause hydronephrosis and lead to renal failure). Early detection with reliable, frontline wet urinalysis testing is essential in the clinical diagnosis and management of urinary tract infections.

Bladder Tumors and Lower Urinary Tract Neoplasia

Lower urinary tract neoplasia is relatively common: 90% of these cases are of uroepithelial origin. Primary lower urinary tract neoplasia includes ureteral, bladder, and urethral tumors. The majority of these tumors present in the bladder. It is estimated that each year approximately 52,000 new cases of bladder cancer will be diagnosed in the United States, causing 95,000 deaths [Schumann 1995]. When detected at an early stage, the 5-year survival rate for bladder cancer is 90%.

Hematuria and Urothelial Tumors

Hematuria is the most common clinical symptom; it is often intermittent, ranging from gross hematuria to microhematuria [Shenoy 1985]. Asymptomatic microhematuria is present in 13% of the general population. We studied the frequency of hematuria in 82 patients with urothelial neoplasia [Schumann 1995]. Gross hema-

turia was noted in only 10% and was not observed in patients with urothelial carcinoma in situ (the pathologic stage before tumor invasion). It appears that there is no "safe level" of microhematuria. In one specialized cytodiagnostic urinalysis laboratory, we have evaluated over 300,000 urine specimens and have found in patients with urothelial neoplasia that 70% were dipstick-positive for hematuria. Microscopic examination of urine sediment is more sensitive than reagent-strip testing for the detection of microhematuria in patients with urothelial neoplasia. Because hematuria is often an early symptom or sign, the use of urine cytologic testing method is very important in the early detection of urinary tract tumors. The ability of the urinoscopist to recognize epithelial abnormalities, identify mononuclear cells and detect unexplained epithelial fragments in the examination of the wet urinalysis sediment is crucial in triaging those patients that will need more sophisticated urine cytology. These entities in urine sediment can no longer be ignored by the competent frontline urinoscopist. They must be accurately identified and reported to the physicians so further diagnostic testing can be initiated.

Renal Neoplasia

Renal cell carcinoma accounts for 2% to 4% of all adult cancers. The American Cancer Society estimates that more than 26, 000 new cases and over 10,000 deaths will be attributable to this disease, which has a

2:1 prevalence in males between the ages of 50 and 70. While no causal factors have been linked directly to renal carcinoma, chewing tobacco, cigar and pipe smoking, and exposure to cadmium, asbestos, gasoline, and coke-oven products appear to increase the risk of this disease. Renal cell carcinoma is referred to as the internists' tumor because the lesion is often diagnosed by its systemic rather than its urologic manifestations. One or more of the classical symptoms of hematuria, flank pain, and a palpable abdominal mass can be found in only one third of patients, yet twice that number present with microhematuria. Gross hematuria appears in the later stages of the disease after the tumor has grown to considerable size, with invasion and kidney tissue destruction of the collecting systems [Schumann 1995].

Renal cell carcinomas are traditionally diagnosed by intravenous pyelography (IVP) and arteriography, ultrasonography, computed tomography (CT), radionucleotide scan, and fine-needle aspiration of cystic and/or solid areas. Unfortunately, urinalysis is limited in the early detection, diagnosis, and management of renal tumors.

Types of Urinalyses

Currently, *three* types of urinalysis are practiced. They include: (1) *dipstick analysis* for physician offices and patient or individual home testing providing frontline chemical evaluation of the urine; (2) complete *wet urinalysis,* commonly referred to as a *routine, screening* or *basic* urinalysis, which provides both frontline chemical and sediment evaluation for physician offices, clinics, and hospital-based and clinical reference laboratories; (3) *cytodiagnostic urinalysis*, which is a specialized, quantitative, cytologic approach performed by highly skilled urinoscopists and/or medical laboratory directors, pathologists, medical centers, and reference laboratories where the urine sediment evaluation and correlative urine chemistries are performed on Papanicolaou-stained sediment.

Dipstick Urinalysis

Dipstick urinalysis is a frontline, semiquantitative test for the detection and monitoring of chemical and metabolic abnormalities. Diabetic patients often monitor their own disease for signs of glucosuria, ketonuria, proteinuria, and urinary tract infections by home testing of urine. Reagent-strip testing involves the patient more in the monitoring and improvement of his/her clinical condition and can determine when a doctor's visit is necessary.

Wet Urinalysis

Wet urinalysis provides a cost-effective screening and monitoring test for the detection of both chemical and morphological urine sediment disturbances in urine. Wet urinalysis procedures depend on two major components: (1) *macroscopic urinalysis,* or physicochemical determinations (color, clarity, specific gravity, multiparameter reagent-strip or dipstick measurement of several chemical constituents), and (2) *microscopic urinalysis* (bright-field or phase-contrast microscopic examination of urinary sediment for morphologic evidence of hematuria, pyuria, crystalluria, cylindruria, and microorganisms. With experience and use of modern wet urinalysis technology, a urinoscopist can detect many conditions that can then be monitored with this easily performed diagnostic, frontline urine laboratory test.

Cytodiagnostic Urinalysis

Cytodiagnostic urinalysis is a highly specialized medical laboratory test that comprises macroscopic examination, multiparameter chemical reagent-strip determinations, and standardized cytocentrifugation and Papanicolaou-stained urinary sediment examination. It allows identification and differentiation of lymphocytes, neutrophils, eosinophils, cells with viral inclusions, and convoluted and collecting duct renal tubular cells. Cytodiagnostic urinalysis has been developed over the past decade to identify and characterize urine sediment entities in a variety of clinical settings (renal transplant, multiple myeloma, candidiasis, disseminated lymphoma) and is well correlated with clinical diagnoses in a variety of clinical conditions such as bladder cancer, precancerous urinary tract lesions, urinary inflammation, and urinary tract infections. In urinalysis, the most important factors in the diagnosis of glomerular diseases have generally been the presence of dysmorphic erythrocytes, heme-granular casts (blood), and erythrocytic casts, whereas lymphocyturia and increased exfoliation of collecting duct cells have been indicators of renal tubular disorders and acute rejection in renal transplant recipients. Unlike the renal biopsy, cytodiagnostic urinalysis can be repeated daily, is relatively inexpensive, and allows the regression or progression of the renal injury to be monitored [Marcussen 1992].

Changing Times for Urinalysis

In the 1960's, the use of reagent-strip technology for macroscopic urinalysis provided a laboratory solution for a rapid, cost-effective, semi-quantitative method of screening individuals for hematuria and for the functional monitoring of patients with renal or metabolic disorders. Concurrently, interest in microscopic urinalysis declined because of crude methods, lack of automation, poor clinicopathologic correlations, few continuing education activities, and limited quality control and assurance procedures.

Since 1974, laboratory observations and clinical research studies have shown frontline wet urinalysis using conventional bright-field microscopy to be unreliable and insensitive in the detection and monitoring of many renal and lower urinary tract disorders. While technological advances have occurred using multiparameter reagent-strip tests and immunologic methods, the time-consuming microscopic examination of urinary sediment has remained poorly standardized and clinically under used. Urine microscopy was performed with poor visualization and little physician interest and confidence in the laboratory results. In fact, nephrologists and urologists often omitted ordering urinalysis from commercial and hospital-based laboratories, preferring to perform this medical laboratory procedure themselves. It wasn't until the emergence of standardized wet sediment slide systems that sediment interpretation moved back into the laboratory setting. The urinoscopist's ablty to identify the components that determine a normal, abnormal, or indeterminate sediment finding, and its relationship to the diagnosis of the patient, is crucial to providing the medical value of performing a complete frontline wet urinalysis. Due to its limitations, in 1976 the value of Papanicolaou staining of urinary sediment was reviewed. Traditionally used in the field of diagnostic urinary cytology, it was applied to renal transplant patients and compared with renal histopathology (needle biopsies and nephrectomy specimens).

Clinical Objectives of Urinalysis

The clinical laboratory examination of urine involves a variety of procedures or techniques used by different professionals of the medical and/or pathology laboratory. In general, clinical urine laboratory tests must accomplish the following: (A) *screen* asymptomatic individuals for the presence of disease; (B) aid in the establishment of a *diagnosis* in asymptomatic and symptomatic individuals; (C) obtain *prognostic* information in patients with known disease; and (D) *monitor* the efficacy of treatment (**F**1.1). For physicians using wet urinalysis tests, it is important to distinguish the specific clinical uses and to understand fully the

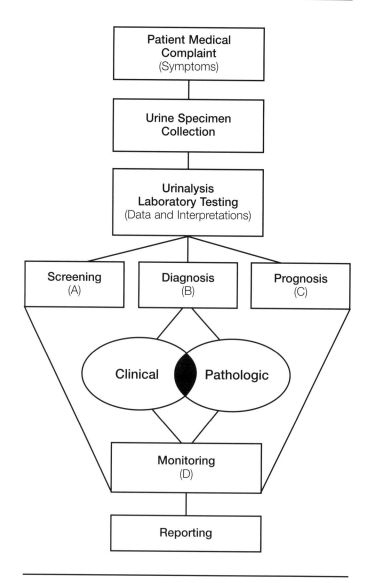

uniquely different types of laboratory information that can be generated by this urine test.

Although cytodiagnostic urinalysis is a diagnostic and confirmatory test, it should not be considered a broad screening or frontline test because it's primary clinical value lies in its early detection and monitoring of various renal and lower urinary tract disorders. Wet urinalysis is a true frontline screening test because it provides both physicochemical and urine sediment data, as well as interpretation and diagnosis of the urine sediment findings.

Frontline Diagnostic Wet Urinalysis

Frontline diagnostic wet urinalysis incorporates technological advances in multiparameter reagent-strip chemical testing, confirmatory chemical methods, and a qualitative and quantitative assessment of urine

Wet Urinalysis

sediment entities. A definitive interpretative statement is based upon an accurate interpretation of urine sediment findings and correlation with urine chemical information. The wet urinalysis interpretation (diagnosis) tells the clinician what chemical and morphologic abnormalities are present in a urine sample and makes appropriate recommendations for confirmation or additional testing.

Basic Components of Diagnostic Wet Urinalysis
The wet urinalysis examination consists of four major components:
1. An adequate patient history
2. A physical examination of the urine sample, including color, clarity (appearance), and specific gravity
3. A chemical examination consisting of a multiparameter reagent-strip testing and confirmatory chemical tests
4. An accurate microscopic urine sediment examination which includes:
    a. A standardized microscopic slide system
    b. Use of the bright-field or phase-contrast microscope
    c. A qualitative and quantitative microscopic examination to identify clinically important urine sediment entities and the systematic evaluation of 10 specific morphologic categories:
        Background
        Erythrocytes
        Leukocytes
        Microorganisms
        Epithelial cells
        Casts
        Lipids
        Epithelial fragments
        Epithelial abnormalities
        Concretions and secretions

Appropriate recommendations for further confirmatory testing such as cytodiagnostic urinalysis and clinical follow-up should be included.

Clinical Utility of Diagnostic Wet Urinalysis
The clinical laboratory examination of urine (urinalysis) can provide useful information on kidney and lower urinary tract and other systemic diseases.

F1.2 **Chain of Events for Optimal Wet Urinalysis Testing**

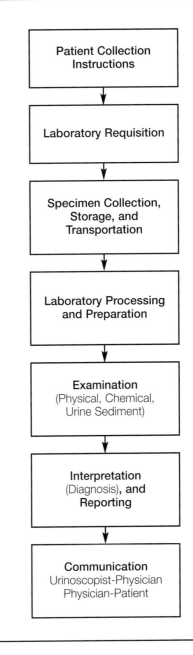

Both structural (anatomical) and functional (physiological) disorders of the kidney and lower urinary tract may be elucidated as well as sequential information about the disorder or disease, its cause, and prognosis. Usually this data can be obtained without pain, danger or distress to the patient. Therefore, properly performed and interpreted wet urinalysis testing will always remain an essential frontline part of clinical medicine even in this rapidly changing health care environment.

The chain of events for optimal testing is illustrated in **F**1.2.

T1.2 provides an explanation of each of the important steps.

Collection Instructions	The foundation of all wet urinalysis testing is the urine specimen. Collection instructions should be provided to the patient in a clear, uncomplicated fashion. Understanding that an improperly collected specimen may result in inconclusive results and/or the necessity of repeat collection will aid in successful specimen collection
Laboratory Requisitions	Each clinical urinalysis laboratory has its own requisition form. The information included on the form is required by a number of healthcare regulatory agencies. The type of specimen, test ordered, patient name, date of birth and other pertinent information must be included on the form.
Specimen Collection, Storage, and Transporation	Instruction on the collection of any urine specimen should be the optimum conditions to be met. If the storage and transportation of specimens will impact the analysis such as the viability of the specimen if stored unfixed, and unrefrigerated, the instructions in the kit should be reinforced through continuous education to the client.
Laboratory Processing and Preparation	The clinical urinalysis laboratory is responsible for ensuring that the information is current. All procedures related to the flow of the urine sample through the laboratory must be included in a procedure manual. The manual must be current and accessible to laboratory personnel.
Wet Urinalysis	Wet urinalysis testing is performed on the proceeded urine samples and is performed by clinical laboratory professionals. Parameters and protocols for the analysis must be established and adhered to in a consistent manner. Continuous quality and assurance programs must be a part of each laboratory procedure and the process for this must be described in the procedure manual.
Interpretation (Diagnosis) **and Reporting**	All urinalysis interpretations (diagnosis) must be documented and the documentation must be available for review for not only future correlations for the patient but for regulatory agencies. Reporting to the physician should include all information used to arrive at an interpretation. This should include the patient and ordering physician information, identification number provided by the laboratory, clinical data, macroscopic and microscopic descriptions, qualitative and quantitative descriptions (with normal/abnormal reference ranges) and the diagnostic interpretation. A pathologist or laboratory director should be available to review abnormal findings.
Physician Communication	Results should be demonstrated to the patient and be supportive to the physician/patient communication regarding patient wellness and/or the need for further testing. The urinoscopist communicates with the physician by report unless the determination has been made that specific diagnoses are to be called in to the physician. Communication of what actions should be taken in patient treatment should be an integral part of all physician communication.

Limitations of Diagnostic Wet Urinalysis

Wet microscopic urinalysis using unstained or stained bright-field microscopy is traditionally used to screen asymptomatic patients exhibiting macroscopic urinalysis abnormalities. Using standardized slide systems and microscopic enhancements such as phase-contrast microscopy, wet urinalysis is useful for early detection of hematuria, renal disorders, and urinary tract infections. However, the following urine sediment findings are difficult to interpret using unstained bright-field microscopy:

▶ *Mononuclear cells: lymphocytes, plasma cells, eosinophils, histiocytes, macrophages, and renal tubular epithelial cells*

▶ *Inclusion-bearing cells: differentiation of virus, drug, and heavy metal induced inclusions*

▶ *Pathologic casts: renal tubular, neutrophilic, eosinophilic, lymphocytic, mixed, bile, fibrin, fungal, and myeloma*

▶ *Abnormal epithelial fragments*

▶ *Premalignant and malignant urothelial cells*

The urinoscopist must understand the limitations of wet unstained sediment analysis and situations that require further confirmation.

Coordination Between Diagnostic Wet Urinalysis and Cytodiagnostic Urinalysis

Over the last 20 years, a coordinated approach to the clinical laboratory examination of urine has been developed to enable the clinician to select the best urinalysis test for a specific clinic need [Schumann 1983]. Wet urinalysis and cytodiagnostic urinalysis are two distinct, complementary clinical laboratory tests for the evaluation of urine. Indications for their use are given in **F**1.3.

Wet urinalysis (left side of the figure) is the best front-line screening procedure for asymptomatic individuals and for patients with signs and symptoms such as hematuria, dysuria, frequency, urgency, and oliguria. Wet urinalysis is also valuable for the rapid assessment of

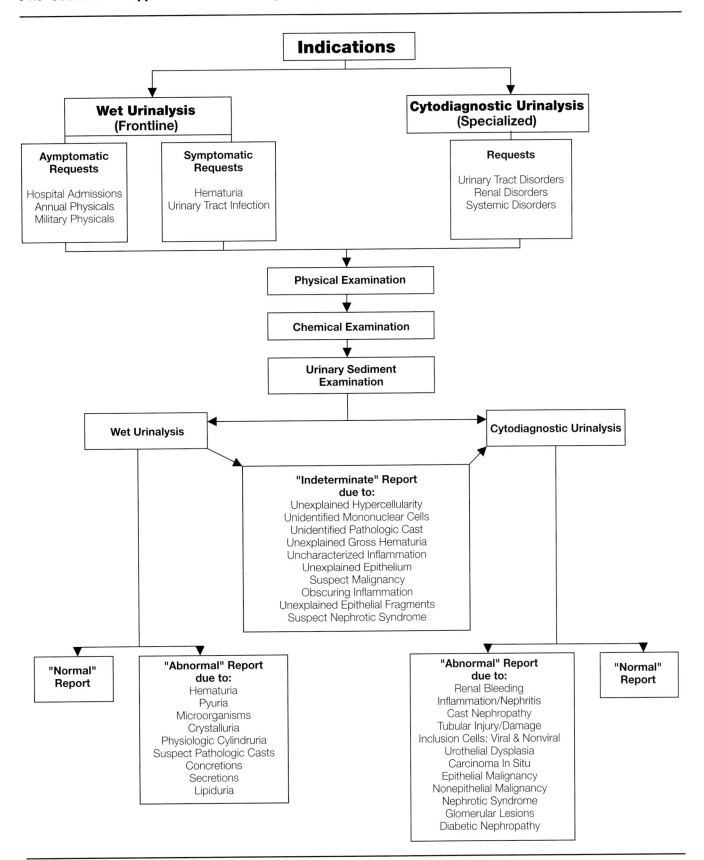

common chemical constituents (protein and glucose, etc.).

Cytodiagnostic urinalysis is valuable in evaluating immunosuppressed patients, in screening individuals with nephrotoxic or carcinogenic exposures, and in diagnosing patients suspected to have kidney and lower urinary tract disorders. In addition, this specialized urine test can often explain indeterminate results of hypercellular samples, by distinguishing specific types of mononuclear cells as hematopoietic, microbiologic, or epithelial (renal or urothelial), and by characterizing the various types of pathologic casts and epithelial fragments. The right side of **F**1.3 lists the information that can be obtained from cytodiagnostic urinalysis.

Several studies have concluded that a bridge between wet urinalysis and cytodiagnostic urinalysis is needed to deal with the common problem of indeterminate results. When correctly instituted, the coordinated approach to the urine sediment examination provides a logical, cost-effective pathway to more sophisticated and costly procedures and technology. It provides reasonable guidance and prevents the premature use of invasive procedures such as a renal biopsy. Additionally laboratory techniques such as microbiologic, immunologic, and histopathologic studies, static and flow cytometry with DNA analysis, electron microscopy, and new molecular biology studies may also be used more effectively.

References

Carlson DA, Statland BE. Automated urinalysis. *Clinics Lab Med* 8:449–461, 1988.

Haber MH. Pisse profecy: A brief history of urinalysis. *Clinics Lab Med* 8:415–430, 1988.

Horowitz PJ, Saladino AJ, Dole JC. Timeliness of urinalysis. A College of American Pathologists Q-Probe study of 340 small hospitals. *Arch Pathol Lab Med* 121:667–671, 1997.

Marcussen N, Schumann JL, Schumann GB, et al. Analysis of cytodiagnostic urinalysis findings in 77 patients with concurrent renal biopsies. *Am J Kid Dis* 20:618–628, 1992.

Schumann GB, Schumann JL, Marcussen N. *Cytodiagnostic Urinalysis of Renal and Lower Urinary Tract Disorders.* New York; Igaku-Shoin, 1995.

Schumann GB, Schumann JL, Schweitzer S. The urine sediment: a coordinated approach. *Lab Management* 21:45–48, 1983.

Shenoy UA. Current assessment of microhematuria and leukocyturia. *Clinics Lab Med* 5:314–329, 1985.

Anatomy and Physiology of the Urinary System

Gross Anatomy and Histology of the Kidneys

The kidneys are located in the mid-upper retroperitoneum on either side of the vertebral column and abdominal portions of the great vessels. The retroperitoneum is a space filled with connective tissue between the musculature of the posterior abdominal wall and the peritoneal lining the abdominal cavity posteriorly. The kidneys do not lie within the abdominal cavity but behind it and are supported within the retroperitoneum by three connective tissue coverings. The kidney is covered by a fibrous capsule that is surrounded by a layer of fat called the *perirenal fat.* The perirenal fat is surrounded by a thin layer of fibrous tissue called the *renal fascia or Gerota's fascia.* While the connective tissue elements in the retroperitoneum are important for support of the kidneys, because this tissue is so loose, it allows for easy spread of renal abscesses which might extend beyond the capsule of the kidney.

Relation of the Kidney to Other Anatomic Organs

Posterior

Both kidneys lie on the posterior abdominal wall musculature. In addition, the superior portions of both kidneys are protected posteriorly by the lower ribs.

Anterior-Right Kidney

Superior pole is covered by the adrenal gland and right lobe of the liver. Medial aspect is covered by the duodenum, the lateral portion is covered by the small bowel and the inferior portion is covered by the colon.

Anterior-Left Kidney

Superior pole is covered by adrenal gland. Superior and lateral portion is covered by the spleen, medial aspect is covered by the stomach, pancreas, and small bowel, and the inferior portion is covered by the colon.

Shape and Size of the Kidney

Adult kidneys normally weigh between 140 and 160 g. The kidneys normally measure 10 cm in length, 5 cm in width, and 2.5 cm in thickness. The kidneys are generally ovoid but are deeply indented along the medial margin where the renal arteries enter the kidney and the renal veins and ureters exit the kidney. This indented region is called the *hilum.*

External Blood Supply and Drainage

The kidneys are supplied by the renal arteries, which arise from the mid-portion of the abdominal aorta. The left renal artery is shorter than the right as the aorta is on the left side of the vertebral column. Thus the right renal artery has to cross the midline behind the inferior vena cava to reach the right kidney. As the renal artery approaches the kidney, it usually splits into five segmental arteries. Three or four of these usually enter the hilum anteriorly, while one or two enter the hilum posteriorly. Each of the five segmental arteries supplies one of five segments of each kidney. Segmental veins analogous to the arteries drain each of the kidney segments and join to form the renal veins. The renal veins join the inferior vena cava. In contrast to the renal arteries, the right renal vein is short

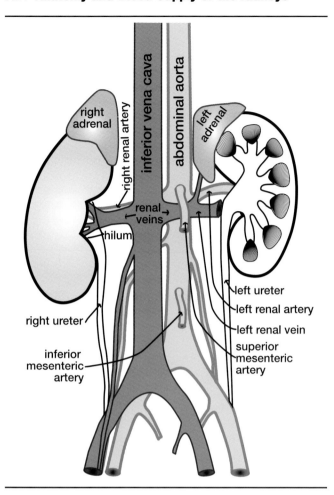

while the left renal vein is longer and has to cross the midline anterior to the aorta to reach the inferior vena cava. The superior mesenteric artery takes off from the aorta anteriorly and crosses directly over the left renal vein. Renal blood supply and drainage are shown in **F**2.1.

Gross Anatomy of the Kidney

The cortex, or outer layer, contains primarily glomeruli and proximal and distal tubules. Medullary rays are faint striations containing collecting tubules, thick ascending limbs of the loop of Henle and terminal portions of proximal tubules.

The medulla or inner layer has two zones. The inner zone (papilla) contains collecting ducts, thin limbs of loop of Henle, loop of Henle, and vasa recta. The outer zone has two stripes. The outer stripe contains mainly the terminal portion of proximal tubule. The inner stripe contains collecting tubules and thick ascending limbs of loop of Henle.

Minor calyces collect urine from collecting tubules piercing the papillae. Seven to 14 minor calyces drain into a major calyx. Two or three major calyces drain into the renal pelvis, which drains into the ureter.

Microanatomy of the Kidney

Internal Blood Flow

Each kidney can be divided into five segments, apical, upper, middle, lower, and posterior each of which is supplied by its own segmental branch of the renal artery. Each segmental artery divides initially giving rise to lobar arteries (**F**2.2). Each segmental lobar artery in turn gives rise to several interlobar arteries which extend into the kidney to the level of the corticomedullary junction. At this junction the interlobar arteries arc and follow the line of the junction and are called *arcuate arteries*. The arcuate arteries give off branches called interlobular arteries. Each interlobular artery gives off small afferent arterioles in a radial fashion. Each afferent arteriole supplies a single glomerulus.

The glomerulus is a ball of capillaries supplied by the afferent arteriole in which the blood is filtered and is drained by the efferent arteriole. Efferent arterioles from glomeruli in the outer cortex will break up and form a capillary plexus that supplies mainly the proximal and distal tubules and the collecting ducts. However, efferent arterioles from glomeruli near the medula (juxtamedullary) supply not only the proximal and distal tubules and collecting ducts, but also branch down into the medulla and form capillary plexi around the loops of Henle and more distal collecting ducts. The branches of the efferent arterioles that supply the medulla in this manner are called the *vasa recta*. The vasa recta play a very important role in the countercurrent exchange mechanism of the kidney.

Venous branches of the vasa recta drain the medulla and venous branches of the capillary plexi of the tubules in the outer cortex drain the cortex. The venous branches join to form interlobular veins. Interlobular veins empty into the arcuate veins which empty into interlobar veins which empty into lobar veins which empty into segmental veins, etc.

Glomeruli

The glomerulus is fed by the afferent arteriole and consists of a complex tuft of capillaries which appears to be divided into up to eight lobules. These lobules have a central connective tissue core called the *mesangium* which supports the capillaries and possibly performs other roles in maintenance of the glomerulus and regulation of blood flow through it. The endothelial cells of the capillaries exhibit pores or fenestrations. The capillary endothelial cells are covered by a basement membrane composed of a collagen-like glycoprotein.

A layer of epithelial cells rests on the capillary basement membrane. These cells have extensions called *foot processes* which rest on the capillary basement membrane and are important in the filtration process.

These epithelial cells form the layer over the capillary tuft of the glomerulus known as the *visceral epithelium.*

The glomerular tuft extends into a capsular space bound by *Bowman's capsule* which is made up of an epithelium and a basement membrane. The epithelium is flattened and continuous with the epithelium overlying the capillary tuft basement membrane and the epithelium lining the proximal tubule. This epithelium is called the *parietal epithelium.* The basement membrane is continuous with the capillary tuft basement membrane and with the basement membrane of the proximal tubule.

The capillary tuft of the glomerulus is drained by the efferent arteriole. The glomerular filtrate exits the glomerular capillary, passes through the capillary basement membrane and foot processes of the visceral epithelium into the capsular space. This *ultrafiltrate* then passes into the proximal convoluted tubule.

At the hilus of the glomerulus between the afferent and efferent arterioles is a structure called the *juxtaglomerular apparatus* consisting of three parts; specialized cells in the wall of the afferent artriole; macula densa which is composed of cells of the part of the distal tubule lying nearest the hilus of the glomerulus; specialized cells located between the macula densa and the cells in a afferent artiole. This structure is intimately involved in sodium metabolism and renin production.

Tubules

Proximal convoluted tubule. Responsible for reabsorption and secretion of various important ions and biochemicals. The tubules consist of two parts (**F**2.2): *convoluted* part (pars convoluta), ramifies around the parent glomerulus and straight part (pars recta), which is the terminal portion of the proximal tubules after it enters the medullary ray.

Lined by a tall cuboidal epithelium with eosinophilic granular cytoplasm and a small round central nucleus, the luminal edge of the cell demonstrates a brush border composed of *microvilli.* The basal portions of the cells in the pars recta exhibit cell membrane infoldings as well. Both the microvilli and infoldings serve to increase surface area for the functions of secretion and reabsorption.

Loop of Henle. The pars recta of the proximal tubule gives way to the thin descending limb of the loop of Henle (**F**2.2), which takes part in the countercurrent mechanism leading to urine concentration. The thin descending and ascending limbs and the loop itself are all of narrow caliber and are lined by a flattened epithelium with few prominent features. The thin limbs and loop lie in close proximity to the vasa recta of the efferent arterioles which also are important in the countercurrent mechanism.

The thick ascending limb of the loop of Henle functions in sodium reabsorption. The ascending loop is present in the medullary rays and is lined by tall cuboidal cells with apical nuclei and no brush border.

F2.2 Diagrammatic Anatomy of a Nephron

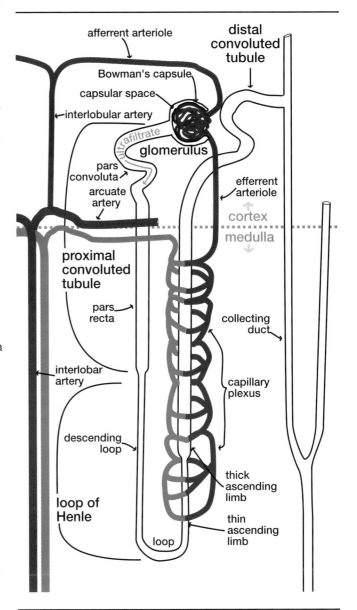

Distal convoluted tubule. The distal convoluted tubule is in sodium and water reabsorption. Short and less convoluted than proximal tubule. Becomes closely associated with the glomerules and forms the macula densa. Lined by pale low cuboidal cells with central or apical nuclei.

Collecting ducts. Transport urine from nephrons to calyces and are responsible for further water reabsorption. They are present in medullary rays and are lined by cuboidal cells with light staining cytoplasm and central nuclei, with no brush border.

Calyces and Renal Pelvis

Collecting tubules empty into minor calyces which in turn empty into major calyces, which in turn empty into the renal pelvis, which in turn empties into the ureters. The anatomy of the calyces and pelvis are demonstrated in

F2.3 Calyces Demonstrated on Cross-Section

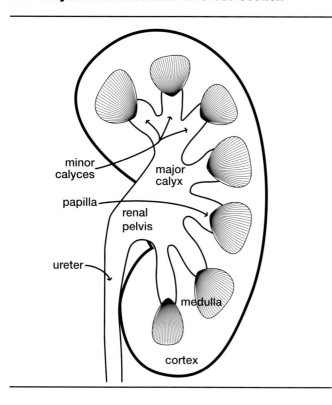

F2.3. Their lining is made up of a transitional epithelium called *urothelium*.

Gross Anatomy and Histology of the Ureters

The ureters are muscular tubes that carry urine from the renal pelvis to the bladder by peristaltic waves. Ureters are approximately 25 cm in length and 9.5 cm in diameter. They are completely retroperitoneal and about ½ abdominal and ½ pelvic. Ureters descend almost vertically along psoas major muscle and join the bladder posteriorly in a region called the *trigone*.

As they enter the bladder, they do so in an oblique fashion. Because of this and the generally contracted state of the bladder muscle, the ureter essentially has a one-way valve at the bladder preventing retrograde flow. In some people this valve is incompetent allowing reflux of urine into the ureters from the bladder, which in turn allows for stasis of urine in the ureters and backflow.

Ureteral Blood Supply

Blood supply to the ureters is from renal arteries, ovarian or testicular arteries, aorta, internal and common iliac, vesical arteries and uterine arteries.

The ureters cross the external iliac arteries anteriorly. In females, the uterine arteries cross the ureters anteriorly in the pelvis. This relationship is vital as any type of uterine surgery can easily lead to damage of the ureter.

The ureter is predisposed to obstruction at two major sites; the ureteropelvic junction where the ureter is slightly narrowed at this point and can be further compromised by renal vessels entering the hilum, leading to stasis; and at its crossing of the external iliac artery, where the ureter is narrowed by the iliac and in a few people can be pronounced, again leading to stasis. The ureters are lined by urothelium.

Anatomy and Histology of the Urinary Bladder

Gross Anatomy

The urinary bladder is a muscular pouch that lies in the superior portion of the pelvis just posterior to the pubic bones and just inferior to the peritoneal floor of the abdominal cavity.

The bladder has four walls, a superior wall, a posterior wall, and two inferolateral walls. The base or posterior wall contains the region of the trigone where the ureters enter superoposteriorly. The anterior most point where the superior wall and inferolateral walls meet is called the apex. At the inferior most point where the posterior and inferolateral walls meet, the bladder narrows to form a neck which enters into the urethra.

The wall of the bladder is composed mainly of the detrusor muscle which consists of three layers of smooth muscle running in three different directions. At the neck of the bladder the detrusor forms the internal sphincter of the bladder which is under involuntary control. As the bladder fills with urine the detrusor muscle stretches but also contracts at the same time increasing pressure in the bladder. At a certain point the pressure will become great enough that the internal sphincter will relax allowing urine to flow if the external sphincter is voluntarily relaxed. If the external sphincter is not relaxed and pressure continues to build, at a certain point a reflex action will occur relaxing the external sphincter. The bladder is lined by urothelium (transitional epithelium).

Anatomy and Histology of the Urethra

Male

The urethra is a channel 15 to 20 cm in length conveying urine from the bladder to the external urethral orifice at the tip of the glans penis. The male urethra is made up of three parts: prostatic, membranous and penile. The prostatic urethra begins at the bladder neck and passes through the prostate a distance of about 3 cm. The bladder neck sits right on top of the prostate. As it passes through the prostate it accepts prostatic secretions and connects to the ejaculatory ducts posteriorly. The prostatic urethra is lined by urothelium.

Membranous urethra extends from the lower pole of the prostate to the bulb of the corpus spongiosum of the penis. This portion of the male urethra is surrounded by the urogenital diaphragm, which contains several small muscles forming the external urethral sphincter. This is skeletal muscle and is under voluntary control. The membranous urethra is lined by stratified or pseudostratified columnar epithelium.

The penile urethra composes most of the urethra. It extends from the bulb of the corpus spongiosum of the penis to the tip of the urethra and is lined by stratified columnar epithelium which gradually gives way to stratified squamous epithelium near the end of the urethra.

Female

The female urethra is a short muscular tube measuring 6 cm in length. From the bladder it passes anteroinferiorly, posterior and then inferior to the symphysis pubis and anterosuperiorly to the vagina. The external urethral orifice is located between the labia minora, anterior to the vaginal orifice and inferoposterior to the clitoris. It also passes through a urogenital diaphragm distally composed of skeletal muscle acting as the external sphincter under voluntary control. The female urethra is lined throughout its course by stratified squamous epithelium.

Four Major Processes in Urine Formation

Ultrafiltration occurs in the glomerulus and is the process of filtering substances from blood plasma. Blood constituents, primarily plasma, which pass through the glomerulus are called the *ultrafiltrate*. Blood cells remain in the bloodstream. The volume of plasma filtered per time unit is called *glomerular filtration* rate (gfr).

Tubular reabsorption involves the return of specific blood constituents (glucose, calcium ions, sodium ions, water) back into the bloodstream by the renal tubular epithelial cells. Creatinine travels through tubules and out of kidney with little alteration. Tubular reabsorption may be relatively complete for constituents such as glucose, amino acids, or variable (water and electrolytes, calcium and sodium).

Active transport requires metabolic energy. Glucose is actively transported from renal tubular cells to the bold. Passive transport involves differences in concentration or electric potential which create gradients across

membranes. Diffusion and osmosis are examples of passive transport mechanisms.

Tubular secretion is the way in which metabolic wastes are removed from the blood by the renal tubular cells and secreted into the lumen of the renal tubule to join the glomerular ultrafiltrate.

Concentration process occurs as water is removed form the ultrafiltrate filtrate by the tubular and collecting duct cells. Antidiuretic hormone (ADH) and aldosterone may be secreted to aid the concentration process.

Pathway of Urine Formation

Blood enters afferent arteriole, leaves by efferent arteriole.

Blood cells and large molecules are unable to pass the glomerular basement membrane.

Electrolytes, glucose, urea, amino acids and water pass glomerular membranes and comprise the glomerular filtrate—essentially the same as plasma minus cells, lipids and proteins.

Proximal tubules involved in active absorption of glucose, electrolytes; water is passively reabsorbed by osmosis.

Descending tubule is permeable to water and is surrounded by interstitium, whose salt concentration increases from cortex to medulla.

Blood vessels in medulla (vase recta) and ascending and descending loops of Henle with tissue around them form a countercurrent exchange for water and salts resulting in concentration of solute in tissue of the medulla. This is final concentration of urine before it leaves the kidney.

Collecting ducts modify the concentration of urine depending on the state of hydration of the individual.

Well hydrated urine leaves the body as dilute urine. If very dilute, effect is water diuresis.

Dehydrated person needs to conserve water. ADH causes collecting duct cells to become permeable to water. Water moves out of collecting duct into the interstitial tissue. In dehydration, water is retained and concentrated urine is voided.

Aldosterone is secreted by adrenal cortex. Aids in sodium reabsorption, antidiuretic affect since water is reabsorbed with sodium.

Collecting ducts of collecting tubules form and empty into the renal pelvis.

Urine is result of concentration of glomerular filtrate. Glomerular filtrate is 1500 L per day.

Dysfunction of any one portion of the kidney can have serious repercussions on the entire system and body.

References

Schweitzer SC. Renal Physiology and Urine Formation Lectures. Medical Laboratory Sciences Program. University of Utah School of Medicine, Salt Lake City, Utah, 1988. Used with permission.

Wet Urinalysis

Specimen Collection, Preservation and Transportation

CHAPTER

3

Types of Transportation and Storage of Containers

Containers

A proper collection container for urine is one that is clean and thoroughly dried before specimens are collected. Disposable collection containers are commercially available for ease in collecting, labeling, storing, transporting, and testing urine specimens. **T**3.1 lists various types of specimens and their utility.

Wet Urinalysis

Glass bottles, disposable wax-coated paper cups, disposable plastic containers with tightly fitting lids are available in a variety of capacities for urine specimen collection. Urinalysis laboratories commonly use capped conical centrifuge tubes of 10–15 mL volumes. Patients usually void into larger containers from which an aliquot of thoroughly mixed urine is transferred. Special pliable sterile and nonsterile polyethylene bags are available for collection of urine from infants and children who have not been toilet trained. The plastic bags are more comfortable than rigid tube containers and are equipped with adhesive backing around the opening to fasten it to the child so that he can void directly into the bag. This technique is also useful for the bedridden patient. With some clear pliable polyethylene containers, an estimate of excreted volume may be established. The bag may be folded and self-sealed for transportation. For 24-hour collections, a tube is attached to the bag and connected to a collection bottle.

T3.1 **Specimens and Their Uses**

Specimen	Urine Chemistry Analysis	Reason for Use
First Morning	Protein	Most concentrated.
	Urine Sediment	Good recovery of cellular constituents and casts.
	Nitrite	Increased time needed for bacteria to metabolize nitrate.
Random or Spot	Wet Routine Urinalysis	Ease and convenience.
2-4 PM	Urobilinogen	Better differentiation of normal and abnormal results.
12-Hour	Addis Sediment Count	Pattern of formed elements is seen better with long collection periods.
24-Hour	Quantitative Chemistry; (Metabolic) Determinations	Overcomes fluctuations in concentration.
Clean-catch; Catheterization; Suprapubic	Microbiologic Studies	Avoids contamination.
Fasting	Glucose	Shows severe disturbances in carbohydrate metabolism.
Postprandial	Glucose	Shows moderate disturbances in carbohydrate metabolism.

24-Hour Urine Collection

The 24-hour urine collection is used to obtain more accurate measurements of total urine protein, glucose,

15

steroids, creatinine, or electrolyte excretion. The urine sample must be collected in a dry, clean, large container and kept refrigerated. Preservatives such as glacial acetic acid, HCL (hydrogen chloride), or boric acid are often added. The 12–24 hour collection is used to assess the progress of disease or efficacy of treatment. This measurement of the rate of excretion of formed elements was first used by Addis in 1948 to study the natural history of glomerulonephritis. A detailed description of the collection method can be found in many textbooks on urine.

Microbiologic Test Kit

Sterile, commercially available kits for the collection of urine to be examined and cultured for microbiologic studies are available. They usually contain either a sterilized glass container or a sterile plastic disposable container, soap-impregnated sponge, alcohol and dry pads along with specimen labels. The container should be equipped with a tightly fitting sterile cap, which is left in position until the actual data of urine collection is recorded.

Noninstrumented Collection Procedures

Voided Urine

First-morning specimen

Because it is concentrated, the first-morning urine specimen is optimal for the microscopic examination of the sediment [Bradley 1979, Kark 1963]. The concentration of solutes and formed elements in the urine varies throughout the patients waking hours depending upon his water intake. Ordinarily, the first-morning urine specimen, voided on rising, is the most concentrated because the patient has not been consuming liquids during the hours of sleep.

Spot specimen

A randomly collected, or *spot specimen*, however, is often more convenient for the patient and is usually acceptable for most screening purposes.

Collection of Urine for Bacteriologic Examination

If the patient has been properly prepared, clean voided urine specimens are generally adequate for culture and subsequent sediment examination. To avoid contamination of the voided specimen by organisms

from areas adjacent to the urethra, the surrounding area must first be thoroughly cleansed. If the patient is instructed to void and then collect midstream urine, organisms normally found in the distal urethra may be cleared prior to collection. There are instances when urethral catheterization or suprapubic aspiration of the bladder is necessary.

Bacteriologic culture should be performed as soon as possible. A refrigerated urine may be cultured for up to 12 hours. Preservatives or fixatives added to the specimen make the sample useless for culture. Once cultures have been performed, however, fixatives are recommended if specimens are to be used for cytologic evalutation. Quantitative cultures should be performed on successive dilutions of urine. The growth of 10^5 colonies/mL is considered to represent a urinary tract infection. Under these standard conditions, growth of not more than 10^3 colonies/mL usually indicates contamination.

Clean-catch Voided Technique

Males

The glans should be adequately exposed and thoroughly cleaned with a mild antiseptic solution. With the foreskin retracted, the midstream urine should be collected in a sterile container after the initial flow of urine has been allowed to escape.

Females

The urethral opening must be plainly exposed and the urine stream directed. The patient should be positioned astride a bedpan or toilet. The attendant, wearing sterile gloves, separates the labia minora (which should remain separated throughout) to expose the urethral orifice. The area surrounding the urinary meatus and the meatus are cleansed with sterile soapy cotton balls. Using sterile water-saturated cotton balls, the area should be rinsed clean. The patient is instructed to void and to allow the initial stream to drain into the bedpan or toilet. The midstream sample is then collected in a sterile container without touching any portion of the perineum with the container. At least 30–100 mL of urine should be obtained.

Wet Urinalysis

For chemical and microscopic urine sediment evaluation, elaborate cleansing procedures are not required, and a clean-catch specimen is usually suitable. If the specimen is likely to be contaminated by vaginal discharge or menstrual blood, precautions must be taken. At times it may be necessary to pack the vagina, especially when examination of the urinary sediment is critical.

Instrumented Collection Procedures

Urethral Catheterization

Urethral catheterization is considered by many to be an unnecessarily dangerous procedure for most individuals because it may cause iatrogenic genitourinary infections and pyelonephritis. Thus, its use is limited. Properly collected, clean voided specimens are preferable for virtually all examinations including bacteriologic cultures [Kunin 1974].

Urethral catheterization is not a recommended method for collecting urine specimens for bacteriologic examination. There are situations, however, in which urethral catheterization is the only reliable way to obtain a suitable specimen: marked obesity, redundant labia in the female, or illness or weakness so severe that the patient is unable to pass a reliable specimen. Kunin describes a detailed procedure for catheterization of males and females [Kunin 1974].

Suprapubic Needle Aspiration

The suprapubic needle aspiration is the method of choice for collection from infants and young children. If clean voided urine obtained in a disposable bag or regular container gives a positive culture, confirmation by suprapubic aspiration is essential for definitive diagnosis prior to institution of specific therapy. Kunin describes a detailed procedure for suprapubic aspirations [Kunin 1974].

Catheterization and Bladder Irrigation

Catheter drainage is more selective than spontaneously voided urine specimens. Irrigation under flouroscopic control, using saline to "barbotage" a suspected bladder lesion, has been proven to significantly improve cell preservation and cellular yield [Tweeddale 1977]. This method utilizes vigorous transcatheter agitation of the bladder by 50–75 mL of normal saline with subsequent removal of the sample for cytologic study. This method has been suggested to yield the optimum cellular sample of bladder epithelium.

Chemical and Cellular Degeneration

Cellular constituents are said to degenerate or change from a higher to a lower or less functionally active form when there is chemical change in the cell or tissue itself. Degenerative changes begin at the cellular level before the living cells of urinary tract are exfoliated into the urine. Cellular maturation and exfoliation is a process in which the younger, basal cells are constantly regenerating and pushing the more mature living cells closer to the surface of the epithelium, where they are eventually exfoliated. Surface epithelium, which is in contact with proteolytic enzymes and bacterial cytolysins in the urine, will begin the process of cellular breakdown before the actual occurrence of exfoliation [Voogt 1977].

Sources of Degeneration

The effect of bacteria upon nonepithelial constituents, epithelial cells, and chemical properties of urine should be recognized. Bacteria use the glucose in urine and the urea-splitting organisms convert urea to ammonia, producing an alkaline urine. If one considers the rate of bacteria multiplication (doubling exponentially every 20 minutes), the urinalysis laboratory must avoid examining any sample that has been heated or left standing at room temperature longer than 4 hours.

Tonicity

Tonicity is a physical property of urine that must be evaluated and considered with respect to staining properties in the microscopic examiniation [Voogt 1977]. Hypertonic and hypotonic solutions produce effects upon cellular matter by changing the water content of the cell. A hypertonic solution causes the cell to shrink in size. A hypotonic solution induces swelling [Palmieri 1977]. The normal specific gravity of urine varies from 1.005 to 1.030, but usually ranges between 1.010 and 1.025. Specific gravity reflects the quantities of dissolved solids such as urea, sodium and chloride. Hypertonic urine specimens contain larger quantities of dissolved solids and have, therefore, a high specific gravity. The detrimental effect of hypertonic urine is appreciated in mild to severe morphologic changes.

Hypotonic "water-like" urine produces a prominent osmotic effect and exaggerated cellular damage. All epithelial constituents increase in size as water crosses the semipermeable cell membranes swelling and eventually bursting the cells. Loss of nuclear segmentation of neutrophilic leukocytes has been reported in hypotonic urine [Palmieri 1977].[4]

Techniques Used to Minimize Degeneration

Refrigeration

If the examination of urine sediment cannot be undertaken within 1–2 hours after collection, precautions must be taken to avoid deterioration of chemical, noncellular, and cellular constituents of the urine sample.

T3.2 **Urine Preservatives**

Method	Advantage	Disadvantage
Refrigeration	For periods of time from 3–6 hours.	For prolonged periods additional preservatives must be used.
Freezing	For specimen transport.	May destroy formed elements.
Toluene	Preserves acetone, diacetic acid, reducing substances, proteins.	Flammable, difficult to separate from specimen.
Thymol	Adequately preserves most constituents.	Not widely used because it yields false positives for proteins with heat and acetic acid test.
Chloroform	Preserves urine for aldosterone levels.	Settles to bottom of containers.
Formaldehyde	Preserves formed elements.	Interferes with glucose evaluation.
Acids		
HCl	Stabilizes steroids, catecholamines, and vanillylmandelic acid.	Fumes and liquid are hazardous, formed elements are destroyed by HCl.
Boric Acid	Preserves chemical and formed elements.	Uric acid may precipitate out with HCl or boric acid.
Preservation Tablet	Preserves urine for dipstick chemical analysis and sediment evaluation when transportation is necessary.	Unsuitable for sodium, potassium, and hormone analysis.
Chlorhexidine	Preserves urine for glucose determination by hexokinase method for up to 6 weeks.	Useful only for glucose preservation.
Sodium carbonate	Preserves porphyrins and urobilinogen.	Interferes with other urine constituents.

Bacteriologic culture should be done as soon as possible after collection. Cultures may be performed within 12 hours after collection if the urine sample is refrigerated. Refrigeration will allow an accurate examination of sediment (including casts, hematopoietic cells, epithelial cells, crystals, concretions, microorganisms, etc.) up to 48 hours after collection. If the specimen cannot be refrigerated, chemical preservatives or fixatives recommended by the clinical laboratory are extremely useful for minimizing degenerative cellular and non-cellular changes.

Chemical Preservatives

Chemical preservatives allow transportation of a urine specimen from home to doctor's office or laboratory and have been used for shipment of specimens by mail across the country. Chemical

T3.3 **Cytologic Techniques Used to Minimize Degeneration**

Type of Fixative	Composition	Recommended Length of Storage	Comments
No fixative added			
Fresh (room temp)		Up to 2 hours	Not bacteriostatic.
Refrigeration		Up to 48 hours	Inexpensive, not bacteriostatic.
Fixative added*			
50-70% EtOH (1:1 specimen/fixative)	50-70%	Several Days	Common cytologic fixative: Preserves cellular material with minimal shrinkage and hardening of cells.
Esposti's fixative (1:1 specimen/fixative)	95% methanol; 5% glacial acetic acid	Several Days	Smears of sediment may be air-dried.
Modified Esposti's acetic acid fixative (5:1 specimen/fixative)	95% EtOH; glacial acetic acid; sodium chloride	Several Days	Smears of sediment may be air-dried.
Saccomanno's fixative (1:1 specimen/fixative)	50% EtOH or isopropyl alcohol; 2% polyethylene glycol (Carbowax**)	Up to 2 weeks	Common cytologic fixative; inexpensive; commercially available.
Mucolexx† (1:1 specimen/fixative)	Polyethylene glycol; Isotonic metallic salt; Formaldehyde; pH buffers	Indefinitely	Minimal cell shrinkage and distortion; not a sterilizing agent; commercially available.

*Refrigeration not required.
**Union Carbide Corp, New York, NY
†Lerner Laboratories, Stamford, CT

preservatives act as antibacterial and antifungal agents. Their primary purpose is preservation for urine chemistry assays. These chemical preservatives affect chemical analyses, and cannot be used for dipstick urinalysis testing. Certain chemical preservatives, ie, thymol and chloroform, have been found to have specific detrimental effects upon the morphologic constituents of urine sediment. There are currently stabilizer or preservation tablets available that do not affect dipstick chemistries or urine sediment evaluation. **T**3.2 lists urine preservatives.

Formalin Fixative

Formalin or a dilute formaldehyde solution has a negative effect on the Papanicoloau and May-Gruenwald-Giemsa stains. Formalin blurs crisp chromatin staining and often interferes with nuclear staining. Formalin is not recommended as a fixative for cytologic evaluation. Should a specimen be received in formalin, a paraffin-embedded hematoxylin and eosin-stained cell block method may be used.

Cytologic Fixative

T3.3 lists the cytologic techniques used to minimize degeneration. The fixative of choice for urine specimens is Saccamanno fixative, which can be made by the laboratory or purchased commercially. Saccamanno fixative contains 50% ethanol (EtOH) or isopropyl alcohol with 2% polyethylene glycol. Equal volumes of urine specimen and fixative will preserve all noncellular and cellular constituents of the urine sample for up to several weeks (even at room temperature).

References

Bradley M, Schumann GB, Ward PCJ: Examination of urine. In Todd-Sanford, *Clinical Diagnosis by Laboratory Methods*, edited by JB Henry, ed 16. Philadelphia; WB Saunders, 1979.

Kark RM, Lawrence JR, Pollack VE, et al: *A Primer of Urinalysis*, ed 2. New York; Harper & Row, 1963.

Kunin CM: Detection, Prevention and Management of Urinary Tract Infections, ed 2. Philadelphia; Lea & Febiger, 1974.

Palmieri LJ, Schumann GB: Osmotic effects on neutrophil segmentation. An in vitro phenomenon. *Acta Cytol* 21:287-289, 1977.

Tweeddale DN: *Urinary Cytology*, Boston; Little, Brown, 1977.

Voogt HJ, Rathert P, Beyer-Boon ME: Urinary cytology. In *Phase Contrast Microscopy and Analysis of Stained Smears*. New York; Springer-Verlag, 1977.

Dipstick Urinalysis and Additional or Confirmatory Urine Chemical Testing

Background

Dipstick urinalysis is a multi-parameter, semi-quantitative test for the detection of specific gravity, pH, leukocyte esterase, nitrite, protein (macroalbumin), glucose, ketones, urobilinogen, bilirubin, and blood (erythrocytes and hemoglobin) in urine. These urine chemical parameters are useful in the detection and management of renal, lower urinary tract, systemic and metabolic disorders [Boeringer Mannheim 1993]. Dipstick or reagent-strip testing consist of chemical-impregnated absorbent pads attached to a plastic strip. A color-producing chemical reaction takes place when the absorbent pad comes in contact with urine. Color reactions are interpreted by comparing the color produced on the pad with a chart supplied by the manufacturer. Three commonly used reagent strips are manufactured under the trade names Multistix™ (Miles Diagnostics, Tarrytown, NY), Chemstrip™ (Roche Diagnostics, Indianapolis, IN) and Rapignost™ (Behring Diagnostics Inc., Sommerville, NJ).

At one time, chemical reagent-strips or dipstick urinalysis determinations were considered examples of state-of-the-art technology. Prior to the development of the first dry chemical dipstick test for glucose in the 1950s, all chemical urine tests were performed individually in test tubes. Reagent-strip technology significantly reduced the time required for testing and reduced costs (eg, reagents and personnel); enhanced test sensitivity and specificity; and reduced the amount of sample required for testing [Brunzel 1994]. The clinical utility, efficacy, advantage, and limitation of dipstick urinalysis require continual review in light of a changing medical technology and a changing healthcare environment.

Clinical Utility

A major variable in dipstick urinalysis testing is the care taken by the clinical laboratory professional when interpreting the color reactions [Bard 1996]. The subjectivity associated with visual discrimination among colors has been alleviated by the development of semi-automated and automatic instrumentation for the standardized reporting of dipsticks [Strasinger 1985]. Clini-Tek™ (Ames Company, Elkart, IN) measures the light reflected from a reagent-strip that has been manually dipped in urine and inserted into the machine. Light reflection from the test pads decreases in proportion to the intensity of color produced by the concentration of the test substance [James 1978].

The Clinilab™ (Ames Company, Elkhart, IN) adds urine, from vials placed in the machine, to the dipsticks, performs the test for specific gravity, and provides printed results. It relies onthe principle of light reflection for chemical reactions and the falling drop method for specific gravity measurement. This urine instrumentation does not improve the chemical methodology of dipsticks, only the reproducibility and color discrimination [Peele 1977].

One instrument that is specifically designed to meet the needs of the high volume urinalysis laboratory is the Boehringer-Mannheim/Hitachi CHEMSTRIP Super UA™ Automated Urine Analyzer (Indianapolis, IN). The Super UA™ is a reflectance photometer with flexible software that standardizes measurements via selective light emitting diodes (LEDs) at various wavelengths and measurement times coordinated with the chemical reaction occurring in the reagent test area. The instrument uses a microprocessor to convert digital readings into concentration values. The reflected light is, therefore, an indirect measurement of the color change reaction [Boehringer Mannheim 1994].

Dipsticks for wet urinalysis are available through hospitals, laboratories, and pharmacies. The chemical dipstick urinalyses are performed in a variety of settings from hospitals, clinical laboratories, physician's office and the patient's bedside. The reagent test strips are used in annual physical examinations, examination for employment, insurance and military service, as monitoring of therapy and as screening in preventative medicine.

Individuals who use dipsticks include members of the healthcare team, doctors, nurses, clinical laboratory professionals, insurance companies, and patients. Dipsticks are valuable in monitoring the treatment of diabetes by multiple daily urine tests for urinary glucose excretion. In addition, using dipstick urinalysis it is possible to detect the early symptoms of three large disease complexes with a single test strip: carbohydrate metabolism abnormalities (glucose), hemolytic disease (blood), hepatobiliary disease (bilirubin and urobilinogen). New considerations for home-testing include hematuria and proteinuria for kidney function. The cost effectiveness of home dipstick urinalysis testing requires further study.

Manual Procedure for Dipstick Urinalysis

1. Dip the reagent test strip (less than 1 second) into a well mixed, fresh urine specimen at room temperature. Make sure all reagent areas are completely immersed.
2. To remove the strip from the urine, draw the edge of the strip along the rim of the specimen container. Tap strip on absorbent paper to remove excess urine. Hold the strip in a horizontal position to prevent reagent run over.
3. Compare the color changes of the test areas to the color blocks on the color chart provided by the manufacturer at the times indicated for obtaining results.

For the manual procedure, the maximum amount of time required to complete one dipstick evaluation is 2 minutes [Boehringer Mannheim 1993].

When choosing a urine reagent strip for dipstick urinalysis be sure that the specificity and sensitivity limits have met your clinical laboratory requirements. Be sure your test strips are specific, ie, that it reacts only to the substance being tested and no other. The sensitivity or concentration of the substance being

sought must be defined for the various medical communities using this technology.

Principles, Specificity, and Sensitivity of Dipstick Urinalysis

The principles and the reporting of results for protein, glucose, ketones, blood, nitrite, leukocyte esterase, bilirubin, urobilinogen, specific gravity and pH are considered in order herein [Boehringer Mannheim 1993, Strasinger 1985, Free 1974, Ross, 1983].

Protein

Dipstick urinalysis relies on protein error via pH indicators is are more sensitive to the presence of albumin than to other proteins. Reagent strips detect only albumin and will not detect abnormal proteins such as immunoglobulins (Bence-Jones protein) found in multiple myeloma or other gammaglobulinopathies. Therefore, it is very important to screen all urines both with reagent strips and precipitation tests such as sulfosalicylic acid test (SSA). SSA will detect all proteins including albumin, glycoproteins and globulins (Bence-Jones). Refer to **T**4.1 for the SSA procedure and **T**4.2 for its interpretation.

Reagent-Strip Tests	Specificity
Albumin (more sensitive)	Sulfosalicylic Acid (SSA)
	All proteins (albumin, globulin, glycoproteins)

Reagent-Strip Tests	Sensitivity
Multistix™	15–30 mg/dL
Chemstrip™	6 mg/dL
Rapignost™	15 mg/dL
Sulfosalicylic Acid Test (SSA)	5–10 mg/dL

Interferences

Any highly pigmented urine can interfere with the color reaction on the test strip, eg, pigments caused by bilirubin and drugs such a phenazopyridin (Pyridium), which give the urine a very bright orange color.

T4.1 Sulfosalicylic Acid Test for Protein

1. Centrifuge 12 mL of urine.
2. Decant supernatant (11 mL) into a 16 x 125-mm test tube.
3. Add 3 mL of a 7% sulfosalicylic acid reagent.
4. Mix tube by inverting twice.
5. Allow to stand for 10 minutes.
6. Invert tube twice and read.*

*Refer to **T**4.2 for SSA grading guidelines.

T4.2 Sulfosalicylic Acid (SSA) Precipitation Grading Guidelines [Brunzel 1994, Schumann 1989]

SSA Result	Physical Inspection (Observations)	Approximate Protein Concentration	Approximate Protein Concentration by Reagent Strip
Negative	No turbidity	<75 mg/L	<5 mg/dL
Trace	Barely perceptible turbidity. Printed material distorted but readable.	200 mg/L	5–20 mg/dL
1+	Distinct turbidity but no distinct granulation. Cannot read printed material.	300–1000 mg/L	30 mg/dL
2+	Granulation, no flocculation.	1000–2500 mg/L	100 mg/dL
3+	Granulation and flocculation.	2500–4500 mg/L	300–500 mg/dL
4+	Large clumps or solid mass.	>4500 mg/L	>500 mg/dL

False-Positive Results

▶ *Highly buffered or alkaline urines*

▶ *Contamination of urine with residues of disinfectants containing ammonium compounds or chlorohexadine*

▶ *Exposure of urine to the reagent strip for a long period*

False-Negative Results

▶ *When proteins other than albumin are present*

Confirmatory Tests

The sulfosalicyclic acid test (SSA) may be used to confirm the presence of protein or when reagent-strip results are in question.

See **T**4.10 for comparison of urine protein dipstick results and confirmatory SSA test results.

Glucose

Reagent test strips are double sequential enzyme reactions based on the use of the enzyme glucose oxidase.

Specificity

All reagent test strips are specific for glucose and will not detect other sugars such as galactose, lactose, fructose, pentose, and sucrose. Detection of these other sugars, with the exception of sucrose, can be clinically significant in pediatric patients. These other sugars can be detected by using a copper reduction test (Clinitest™ Tablet Test, Miles, Inc.) for reducing sugars.

Reagent-Strip Tests	Sensitivity
Multistix™	75–125 mg/dL
Chemstrip™	40 mg/dL
Rapignost™	30 mg/dL
Clinitest™ Tablet Test	250 mg/dL reducing sugar

Interferences

All reagent strips are specific for glucose, therefore most interferences cause either a reduced or false-negative result.

False-Positive Results

▶ *Chlorine bleach or other oxidizing agents*

▶ *Sensitivity is increased with low specific gravity*

▶ *Strips exposed to air by improper storage*

False-Negative Results

▶ *Large concentrations of ascorbic acid (vitamin C) or from drugs such as tetracycline*

▶ *Moderate levels of ketones (> 40 mg/dL in specimens with small amounts of glucose (75–125 mg/dL)*

▶ *Use of sodium fluoride*

▶ *Cold (refrigerated) urines*

Confirmatory Tests

The Clinitest™ Tablet Test (Miles, Inc.) is the confirmatory test of choice and is based on the ability of glucose or any other reducing sugar to convert copper II (cupric ions) to copper I (cuprous ions) in the presence of heat and alkali. The Clinitest™ test may be performed as either a 5-drop or a 2-drop method. Refer to the procedure in **T**4.3.

Interferences

Tablets must be properly stored and protected from moisture. Inspect tablet for any color change (dark blue or blackish) and do not use if they are not spotted bluish-white in color. The discolored tablets will not provide reliable results.

T4.3 Procedure for Clinitest™ Tablet Test

5-Drop Method

1. Place 5 drips of urine in 15 x 85 mm test tube and add 10 drops of water.
2. Add one Clinitest™ tablet and watch while boiling takes place. DO NOT SHAKE TUBE.
3. Wait 15 seconds after boiling stops, then shake tube gently, and compare the color change to the color scale supplied by manufacturer.
4. WARNING: While solution is boiling, watch if solution passes through orange to a dark shade of greenish-brown. This indicates that the sugar concentration is greater than 2.0 g/dL without reference to the color scale. This is called the "pass-through phenomenon".

2-Drop Method

1. Place 2 drops of urine in 15 x 85 mm test tube and add 10 drops of water.
2. Add one Clinitest™ tablet and watch while boiling takes place. DO NOT SHAKE THE TUBE.
3. Wait 15 seconds after boiling stops, then shake tube gently, and compare the color change to the color scale supplied by manufacturer.
4. WARNING: As with the 5-drop method, watch for the presence of the "pass-through phenomenon".

False-Positive Results

▶ *Large quantity of ascorbic acid (Vitamin C)*

▶ *Specimens that have low specific gravity and contain glucose*

▶ *Large quantities of nalidixic acid, cephalosporins and probenecid*

False-Negative Results

▶ *Shaking tube before the 15-second waiting period after boiling*

▶ *Radiographic contrast media*

Ketones

Reagent test strips are based on Legal's test, a color reaction with sodium nitroprusside in the presence of an alkaline medium, acetoacetic acid will react with sodium nitroprusside to produce a purple color. The reagent test strips are most sensitive to the ketone bodies of acetoacetic acid and acetone.

Reagent-Strip Tests	Specificity	Sensitivity
Multistix™	Acetoacetic Acid	5–10 mg/dL
Chemstrip™	Acetoacetic Acid	9 mg/dL
	Acetone	70 mg/dL
Rapignost™	Acetoacetic Acid	>5 mg/dL
	Acetone	50 mg/dL
Acetest™ Tablet Test	Acetoacetic Acid	5–10 mg/dL
	Acetone	20–25 mg/dL

Interferences

The presence of abnormally colored urine due to various pigments, drugs, or other substances can cause either false-positive or false-negative results.

False-Positive Results

▶ *Urines containing phthaleins (bromsulphthalein, phenosulfonphthalein)*

▶ *Urines containing large amounts of phenylketones*

▶ *High specific gravity*

▶ *Large quantities of levodopa metabolites*

▶ *Compounds containing sulfhydryl groups such as Mesna or Mucomyst*

False-Negative Results

▶ *Improperly stored specimens because of the conversion of acetoacetic acid to acetone*

Confirmatory Test

A tablet test (Acetest™, Miles Diagnostics) tests for acetoacetic acid and acetone. It can be used not only for urine, but for whole blood, serum or plasma.

Blood Hemoglobin and Myoglobin

Tests utilize the peroxidase activity of the heme portion or myoglobin to catalyze a reaction between hydrogen peroxide and *o*-toluidine to produce blue. Reagent strips are equally sensitive to both hemoglobin and myoglobin. In order for the reaction to occur, the red blood cells must come in contact with the reagent strip, lyse, and produce a color change. Urine must be well mixed when tested or a false-negative result will occur, because the intact red blood cells will settle to the bottom of the test tube and will not come in contact with the reagent strip; hence, cells will not be able to lyse.

Reagent-Strip Tests	Sensitivity
Multistix™	0.015–0.062 mg/dL (Equivalent to 5–10 Ery/μL)
Chemstrip™	5 Ery/μL or hemoglobin Corresponding to 10 Ery/μL
Rapignost™	0.015–0.03 mg free hemoglobin/dL urine (Equivalent to 5–10 Ery/μL)

False-Positive Results

▶ *Cleaning agents such as chlorine bleach*

▶ *Microbial peroxidase activity associated with urinary tract infections*

▶ *Menstrual blood*

Wet Urinalysis

24

False-Negative Results

▶ *Ascorbic acid (Vitamin C) > 25 mg/dL*

▶ *Unmixed urine where the intact red cells have settled to the bottom of the tube*

▶ *Elevated specific gravity*

▶ *Elevated protein levels may reduce the lysis of red cells*

▶ *Use of formalin as a preservative*

▶ *Large amounts of nitrite*

▶ *Antihypertensive drug Captopril*

Warning: Ascorbic acid (Vitamin C) remains a potential problem to all reagent strips and causes a false-negative or delayed results. Interference by ascorbic acid is suspected when the reagent strip results are negative yet red cells are seen microscopically or the urine's appearance suggests hematuria.

Confirmatory Test
    Microscopic examination of urine

Additional Test(s)
    Test for ascorbic acid if reagent-strip test for blood is negative, but red cells are seen during microscopic examination.

Nitrite
    The reagent strips are based on the principal of the ability of certain bacteria (not all) that are present in the urinary tract to convert nitrate (a normal urine constituent) to nitrite. Most gram-negative bacteria will cause a positive result. A disadvantage of this test is that the urine must remain in the bladder for at least 4 hours for nitrate to convert to nitrite. The optimum specimen would then have to be the first-morning void or a specimen collected at least 4 hours after the void. This can be difficult for the patient suffering from a urinary tract infection since one of the common symptoms is frequency. The test is specific for nitrite and can be helpful if used in combination with other reagent-strip constituents such as leukocyte esterase to diagnose a urinary tract infection. Definitive diagnosis of a urinary tract infection needs to be confirmed with a microscopic evaluation as well as a microbiological workup. Results are reported either as positive or negative, and the intensity of the color does not indicate severity of bacterial infection.

Reagent-Strip Test	Sensitivity
Multistix™	0.06 to 0.1 mg/dL nitrite ion
Chemstrip™	0.05 mg/dL nitrite ion
Rapignost™	0.05 to 0.1 mg/dL nitrite ion

False-Positive Results

▶ *Bacterial contamination from an improperly collected specimen*

▶ *Medication such as phenaxopyridine*

▶ *Dyes that color urine red*

False Negative Results

▶ *Insufficient incubation of urine in bladder for conversion of nitrate to nitrite*

▶ *Insufficient dietary nitrate present in urine to allow conversion of nitrate to nitrite*

▶ *Starvation, fasting or intravenous feeding all yield a false-negative result.*

▶ *Ascorbic acid (25 mg/dL)*

▶ *Urine with low pH (>6)*

Warning: If reagent-strip test is negative this does not mean the patient is infection-free. There are some bacteria, especially the gram-positive enterococci, and yeast that do not cause a positive reaction; therefore it is imperative that the urine be examined microscopically to rule out a bacterial or yeast infection.

Confirmatory Tests
Microscopic evaluation of urine sediment
Urine culture

Leukocyte Esterase
    Reagent-strip tests for leukocyte esterase are used as another means for detecting urinary tract infections and are specific for esterase that is present in granulocytic leukocytes (PMNs) or neutrophils, monocytes, eosinophils, and basophils). The reagent strip will detect either lysed or intact cells present in the urine. There are other inflammatory conditions that can exist in the urinary tract besides an infection, therefore viewing the urine microscopically becomes very important as a means to rule-out other conditions.

Reagent-Strip Test	Sensitivity
Multistix™	5–15 cells/HPF
Chemstrip™	10–25 cells/HPF
Rapignost™	10–25 cells/HPF

False-Positive Results

▶ *Chlorine bleach*

▶ *Formalin preservation*

- *Elevated glucose levels (>3 g/dL)*

- *High specific gravity*

- *High levels of albumin (500 mg/dL)*

- *Antibiotics such as cephalexin, cephalothin, tetracycline, gentamicin*

- *Large amounts of ascorbic acid*

Confirmatory Tests
Microscopic evaluation of urinary sediment

Bilirubin

Tests for urinary bilirubin are important in detecting liver disease and in determining the cause of clinical jaundice. Reagent strips detect both direct and indirect bilirubin and are based on a diazo reaction in an acid medium producing pink to red-violet, which color is directly proportional to the total bilirubin present.

Reagent Strip Test	Sensitivity
Multistix™	0.4–0.8 mg/dL
Chemstrip™	0.5 mg/dL
Rapignost™	0.5 mg/dL
Ictotest™ Tablet Test	0.05–0.1 mg/dL

Interferences

Since the reagent strip tests are not as sensitive for bilirubin and sometimes difficult to read, it is recommended that Ictotest Tablet Test be performed on all positive reagent strip tests and any urine of patients suspected of having liver disease.

False-Positive Results

- *Drugs such as phenothiazine, chlorpromazine, pyridium, perenium*

- *Bacterial overgrowth*

False-Negative Results

- *Exposure to light will oxidize the bilirubin*

- *High concentration of ascorbic acid (25 mg/dL)*

- *Elevated nitrite concentration as seen in urinary tract infections*

Confirmatory Tests

Ictotest Tablet Test (Miles Diagnostics, Tarrytown, NY) is the test of choice because its sensitivity level is greater than the reagent strips. All urines should be

T4.4 **Ictotest™ Tablet Test for Bilirubin**

1. Place 10 drops of urine on either side of the special absorbent test mat.
2. Place Ictotest™ tablet in center of mat. DO NOT TOUCH TABLET WITH HANDS.
3. Place 1 drop of water onto tablet. Wait 5 seconds and place a second drop of water onto tablet so water runs off tablet onto the mat.
4. At 60 seconds observe mat around or under tablet for a blue to purple color.
5. Report as positive or negative.

tested by this method, even when a positive dipstick result does not occur, whenever the patient has a history of liver problems or is suspicious for disease. Interferences are the same as those for reagent strips. Refer to procedure for Ictotest in **T**4.4.

Urobilinogen

Urobilinogen, like bilirubin, is associated with liver disease and dysfunction. One of the first functions lost when the liver is damaged is the ability of the liver to remove urobilinogen from the blood and re-excrete it into the intestines.

The principle of the reagent strip test for urobilinogen varies with the different manufacturers. Most employ the Ehrlich's aldehyde reaction in which urobilinogen and porphobilinogen react with *p*-dimethyl-aminobenzaldehyde in concentrated HCl acid to form a cherry-red color. The Multistix™ reagent strip uses this principle so a positive reaction indicates the presence of urobilinogen and/or porphobilinogen.

Chemstrip™ and Rapignost™ reagent strips use a different principle. They use a diazo reaction where urobilinogen reacts in an acid medium to form a red azo dye. The strips react to both urobilinogen and stercobilinogen.

Reagent Test Strips	Specificity	Sensitivity
Multistix™	Urobilinogen	0.2 mg/dL
Chemstrip™	Urobilinogen	0.4 mg/dL
Rapignost™	Urobilinogen	1 mg/dL

Interferences

All strips are affected by highly colored pigmented urines caused by azo dyes or their metabolites

False-Positive Results

- *Substances such as sulfonamides, procaine, p-amino-salicyclic acid, and 5-hydroxyindolacetic acid react with Multistix™ reagent strips*

- *Methyldopa*

Wet Urinalysis

► *Serenium, phenazopyridium, nitrofurantoin, riboflavin and* p-*aminobenzoic acid react with all reagent strips*

► *Multistix™ reagent strips are affected by increased temperatures of urine (body temperature)*

False-Negative Results

► *Specimen exposed to light or left at room temperature for more than 1 hour*

► *Formalin preservation*

► *Chemstrip™ and Rapignost™ strips are affected by the presence of ascorbic acid and nitrite*

Confirmatory Tests

The Watson-Schwartz test is a qualitative test that uses the Ehrlich's aldehyde reaction for detection of urobilinogen, porphobilinogen, and any other Ehrlich-reactive compounds. The test involves extraction with both chloroform and butanol producing a pink color. Urobilinogen turns both chloroform and butanol to pink and porphobilinogen leaves both colorless. Precautions must be taken in performing this test due to the carcinogenic properties of chloroform.

Specific Gravity

Specific gravity is the measure of the state of hydration of the patient. If the kidney loses its ability to concentrate or dilute the urine, the specific gravity will remain fixed at about 1.010. The normal kidney can produce a specific gravity ranging from 1.003 to 1.035. Normal specific gravity is the actual measurement of sodium, potassium, chloride, and urea content of the urine. Although normal specific gravity can range from 1.001 to 1.035, it usually ranges between 1.016 to 1.022 in adults with normal fluid intake.

The Multistix™ and Chemstrip™ reagent strips have a test area for specific gravity. Rapignost™ does not. The reagent strips are based on the pka change of certain pretreated polyelectrolytes in relation to the ionic concentration of urine. Readings are made at 0.005 intervals and range from 1.000 to 1.030 and compared to a color chart.

Specificity

Reagent strips measure only ionizable substances.

False-Positive Values

► *Moderate levels of protein*

► *Ketone bodies may elevate strips*

False-Negative Values

► *Highly buffered alkaline urines*

► *Urea concentraton >1 g/dL*

Confirmatory Tests

The use of a refractometer and/or urinometer correlates to within 0.005 of the reagent strips. The fundamental difference between the reagent strips and the urinometer or refractometer is the latter measures any dissolved substances present in the urine. Therefore, the presence of nonionizable substances such as glucose, radiographic dyes, and certain antibiotics can cause false-positive values.

pH

Reagent test strips measure the concentration of free hydrogen by using a double indicator system that consists of methyl red and bromthymol blue. The pH ranges from 5 to 9.

Interferences

There are no known interferences that affect the pH of the urine. Falsely elevated results occur only if the urine is left standing at room temperature for an extended period of time, allowing bacteria to grow within the specimen.

Confirmatory Tests

A pH meter may be used for a more accurate measurement.

Generalized Limitations (Confounders) of Dipstick Urinalysis

False-Positive Results

► *Excess urine on the stick can produce a run over between chemicals on adjacent pads.*

► *A dipstick interference is the masking of color reaction by the orange pigment present in the persons taking Pyridium compounds.*

► *Protein readings can occur if the urine collection bottle contains residues of certain disinfectants composed of quaternary ammonium compounds.*

► *The presence of prostatic and seminal vesicle secretions can give a false positive for protein*

► *The color of urine affects dipstick results*

False-Negative Results

▶ *Lymphocytes are not detected on the dipstick*

▶ *Eosinophils, monocytes/histiocytes, and macrophages are not detected on the dipstick*

▶ *Negative nitrite test does not rule out bacteria*

▶ *It is more difficult to discriminate the colors indicating the lower blood glucose values.*

▶ *The dipstick test cannot determine the absence of urobilinogen, which is significant in biliary obstructions.*

Reliability of Dipstick Urinalysis

A study done by Bonnardeaux et al (1994) on the reliability of dipstick urinalysis found that dipstick reading is an unreliable indicator of what will be seen on the microscopy with dipstick positive urines. The study found poor correlation with positive urines and microscopic findings due to the number of false positives and false negatives for **erythrocytes** (RBCs) and **leukocytes** (PMNs). Sensitivities were 75.3% and 81.0% and specificities were 88.6% and 64.3% for erythrocytes and leukocytes, respectively. Increasing the dipstick cutoff point improved sensitivity but lowered specificity. Also, it is likely that many of the false results are due to poor analytical or reading technique. It may be some time before existing attitudes towards urine testing using reagent strips can be altered to reflect the complexity of a seemingly simple analysis [White 1995].

According to the US Preventive Services Task Force (1989) for the detection of hematuria, the specificity of dipstick urinalysis is 65% to 99.3% when microscopic hematuria is used as a gold standard. The positive predictive value of a positive heme dipstick is 0% to 2% for significant disease, and 6% to 58% for possible significant disease.

T4.5 Types of Specimens for Dipstick Urinalysis

Type of Specimen	Qualities	Good for
First morning	Most concentrated; Bladder incubation.	Nitrite; Protein; Microscopic urinalysis (urine sediment examination).
Random	Most common and convenient.	Chemical screen; Microscopic urinalysis (urine sediment examination)
Second voided	Formed elements intact.	Blood; Glucose.
Postprandial	Collected after meal.	Glucose; 2-hour volume good for urobilinogen; 24-hour volume good for "true" chemical quantitative results.

T4.6 Causes of the Changes in the Color of Urine

Color	Cause
Red or pink	Hematuria; Hemoglobinuria; Myoglobinuria; Porphyrinuria; Phenacetin
Yellow-orange	Rhubarb; Pyridine; Rifampicin; Bilirubin; Phenacetin; Senna; Pyridium
Yellow-green	Riboflavin; Thymol
Brown	Bilirubin; Urobilin; Homogentistic acid; Carotene; Nitrite; Chloroquine; Aniline; Rhubarb
Green	Biliverdin; Santonin; Chlorophyll
Blue	Methylene blue; Indigo blue
Black	Hemoglobinuria; Alcaptonuria
Darkening upon standing	Alcaptonuria; Melanogen; Serotonin; Methyldopa: Porphyrin; Phenacetin

T4.7 Ranges for Urinary Reagent Strips [Strasinger 1985, Ross 1983, Brunzel 1994]

Test Parameters	Normal Reference Range	Abnormal Range
pH	4.7 to 7.8	>7.8
Protein (Macroalbumin)	<14 mg/dL	>14
Glucose	<20 mg/dL	>20 mg/dL
Ketones	Negative	Positive
Bilirubin	Negative	Positive
Blood (Heme)	Negative	Positive
Nitrite	Negative	Positive
Leukocyte Esterase	Negative (10 WBCs/µL)	20 WBCs/µL
Urobilinogen	<1 mg/dL	> 1 mg/dL
Specific Gravity	1.001 to 1.030	>1.030

T4.8 Sensitivity and Specificity of Chemstrip™ Reagent Strips in 90% of Urines Tested

Test Parameters	Sensitivty	Specificity
pH	5.0 to 9.0 in 1.0 increments	No interference known
Protein	6.0 mg/dL in 90%	Most sensitive to albumin
Glucose	40 mg/dL in 90%	Specific for glucose
Ketones	9.0 mg/dL acetoacetate and 70 mg/dL acetone	Does not detect β-hydroxybutyrate
Bilirubin	0.5 mg/dL conjugated bilirubin	Specific for bilirubin
Blood (Heme)	0.02–0.03 mg/dL Hgb	Equally specific for hemoglobin and myoglobin
Nitrite	0.05 mg/dL nitrite ion	Specific for nitrite
Leukocyte Esterase	10 WBC/µL	Detects only granulocytic leukocytes
Urobilinogen	0.4 mg/dL	Reactivity increases with temp, (optimum 22–26°C
Specific Gravity	1.000 to 1.030	Detects only ionic solutions

Test Parameters	False-Positive	False-Negative
pH		
Protein (Macroalbumin)	Highly buffered or alkaline urine pH ; Skin cleansers containing chlorhexidine.	Presence of protein other than albumin; High salt concentrations.
Glucose	Strong oxidizing agents; Chlorine bleach.	Ascorbic acid (>50 mg/dL); Improperly stored specimen; Use of sodium flouride as a preservative; High specific gravity.
Ketones	Compounds with free sulfhydryl groups; Highly pigmented urines.	Volatilization and bacterial breakdown.
Bilirubin	Drug-induced color changes; Large amounts of chlorpromazine	Ascorbic acid (>25 mg/dL); High nitrite concentration; Improper storage.
Blood	Menstrual contamination; Microbial peroxidases; Strong oxidizing agents.	High nitrite (10 mg/dL reduces strip reactivity; Ascorbic acid interference; Elevated protein and specific gravity; Urine not mixed well.
Nitrite	Phenazopyridine; Beets: Improper storage.	Ascorbic acid (25 mg/dL) Factors that inhibit nitrite formation; Urine not retained in bladder for a minimum of 4 hours.
Leukocyte Esterase	Phenazopyridine; Beets; Vaginal contamination.	Lymphocytes not detected; Increased glucose (>3 g/dL); protein (>500 mg/dL); High specific gravity; Cephalosporins; gentamicin; High levels of oxalic acid.
Urobilinogen	Phenazopyridine; Beets.	Formalin (>200 mg/dL); Oxidation to urobilin.
Specific Gravity	Falsely high due to protein (100 to 500 mg/dL; Lactic acids and ketones.	Falsely low due to glucose and urea concentration >10 g/dL; pH >6.5, add 0.005.

For the detection of proteinuria, dipstick urinalysis has a sensitivity and specificity of 95% to 99%. Proteinuria may result from acute illness, exposure to cold, exercise, prostatic secretions, and cells in the urine. The positive predictive value if 0.0% to 1.4% (data obtained from young study populations with low prevalence). The positive predictive value of dipstick urinalysis is too low to justify screening for proteinuria and hematuria, but this may not be the case among the elderly, who have increased risk of urinary tract cancer.

T4.10 **Comparison and Implications of Proteinuria Detected by a Dipstick Urinalysis Test and Confirmatory Sulfosalicylic Acid Test**

Dipstick Result	SSA Result	Implications
Negative	Negative	No proteinuria.
Positive	Positive	Proteinuria.
Negative	Positive	Presence of Bence-Jones (Multiple myeloma); Heavy-chain or other non albumin proteins
Positive	Negative	Drug interference or pH of urine
Positive	Negative	Pathologic concentration of protein is low

Types of Specimens for Dipstick Urinalysis

T4.5 lists the various types of urine specimens for dipstick urinalysis performed in the clinical laboratory. It is the clinical laboratory's responsibility to inform patients and physicians of the optimal specimen required for the specific laboratory assay. **T**4.6 gives causes for the changes in color of urine. Knowledge of reason for these color changes is helpful in explaining to patients the source of the aberration.

Sensitivity and Specificity of Urinary Reagent Test Strips

The ranges for urinary reagent strips are presented in **T**4.7. The urinalysis laboratory should know the sensitivity and specificity of various regent strip methods. Following is the sensitivity and specificity for Chemstrip™ (BMC) reagent strips in **T**4.8. The sensitivity of urinalysis, testing usually increase with multiple or sequential testing **T**4.9 summarizes the clinical laboratory implication of false-positive and false negative reactions in dipstick urinalysis.

Confirmatory Tests and Implications

A confirmatory test detects the same substance with either greater sensitivity or specificity or by utilizing a different reaction to detect that substance. Commonly used confirmatory tests include sulfosalicylic acid (SSA) for proteinuria (**T**4.10),

Ictotest™ for bilirubinuria (**T**4.11) and Clinitest™ for glucosuria (**T**4.12).

Clinical Significance of Positive Reactions

The dipstick test for blood is based on the detection of hemoglobin. Hemoglobin or heme is present in both blood and myoglobin. The screening test for myoglobin is illustrated in **F**4.1. **T**4.13 demonstrates the various reasons for a positive result for blood or myoglobin.

T4.14 lists clinical implications for positive dipstick urinalysis test results. **T**4.15 provides information on dipstick urinalysis results in conjunction with physician or nursing actions that should be taken.

Quality Control and Quality Assurance

The development of quality assurance program for urinalysis has lagged behind other areas of the laboratory. The major errors in urine testing are the following:

▶ *Failure to test a fresh specimen*

▶ *Inadequate specimen collection*

▶ *Use of unclean containers*

▶ *Inadequate care of specimen*

▶ *Failure to adequately mix sample*

▶ *Improper recording of information and test results*

▶ *Poor or inconsistent technique in using the dipstick*

▶ *Inadequate understanding of interfering substances*

▶ *Incomplete training of personnel*

Quality Assurance Procedures

▶ *Specimen identification*

▶ *Specimen handling*

▶ *Written procedures*

▶ *Provide continuing education on dipstick urinalysis*

T4.11 **Possible Causes of Discrepancy Between Bilirubinuria and Ictotest**

Dipstick Result	SSA Result	Implications
Positive	Negative	Metabolite of pyridium gives bright red-orange colors which mask the reaction of small amounts of bilirubin.
Positive	Negative	Elevated concentrations of urobilinogen produce atypical orange colors.
Negative	Positive	False-positive Ictotest due to large amounts of Chlorpromazine™ or metabolites of Lodine®

T4.12 **Possible Causes of Discrepancy Between Dipstick Glucosuria and Confirmatory Clinitest Reducing Substances**

Dipstick Result	Clinitest Result	Implications
Positive	Negative	Low concentrations of glucose present; Clinitest tablets defective (outdated)
Negative	Positive	Other reducing substances present; Reagent strip interference (high specific gravity, low temperature)

F4.1 **Confirmatory Test for Myoglobin**

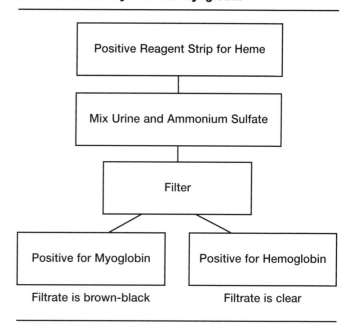

T4.13 **Positive Results for Blood or Myoglobin**

Sources	Visual Inspection (Color of Urine)	Dipstick Urinalysis	Microscopic Urinalysis (Presence of RBCs)	Clinical Condition
Blood	Red	Positive	Positive	Hematuria
Myoglobin	Red	Positive	Negative	Crushing Injury
Food Coloring	Red	Positive	Negative	Food History

T4.14 Clinical Significance of Positive Dipstick Urinalysis Tests

Positive Dipstick Test	Implications
Protein (Macro-albuminuria)	Glomerular membrane damage: Renal disese; Prostatic secretions: Seminal vesicle contaminants.
Glucose	Diabetes mellitus; Impaired tubular injury damages and reabsorption (renal glucosuria).
Ketone	Diabetes mellitus; Diabetic acidosis; Starvation; Excessive carbohydrate loss.
Blood (Heme)	Hematuria; Stress; Strenuous exercise; Trauma: Infection; Stones; Renal injury, damage or disease.
Bilirubin	Hepatitis; Cirrhosis; Biliary obstruction.
Nitrite	Cystitis; Pyelonephritis.
Leukocytes (Esterasuria)	Urinary tract infection (UTI); Inflammation.
Abnormal pH	Affects kidneys' inability to secrete or to reabsorb acid or base.
Urobilinogen	Liver disease; Hemolytic disorders.
Abnormal Specific Gravity (SG)	Low SG = Loss of renal tubular concentrating ability; (Diabetes insipidus). High SG = Adrenal insufficiency; Hepatic disease; Congestive heart failure.

T4.15 Positive Dipstick Urinalysis Results Requiring Physician or Nursing Action

Dipstick Urinalysis and Confirmation Parameter	Action
Blood	Perform wet microscopic urinalysis
Glucose	Perform wet microscopic urinalysis; Rule out Diabetes mellitus; Use cytodiagnostic urinalysis to rule out diabetic nephropathy, infection, renal tubular injury, and renal glucosuria.
Ketones	Rule out acidosis
Protein	Perform wet microscopic urinalysis to exclude renal disorders
Protein and SSA	Use cytodiagnostic urinalysis to rule out glomerular disease or nephrotic syndrome; Perform renal function test
Bilirubin and Ictotest	Perform cytodiagnostic urinalysis to determine renal injury and/or damage; Perform liver function test
Leukocytes Esterase	Perform wet microscopic urinalysis to exclude inflammation and infection
WBC and Nitrite	Perform wet microscopic urinalysis to rule out urinary infection; Urinary microbiologic studies
Urobilinogen	Liver function tests

Quality Control for Dipstick Urinalysis

▶ *Bottles should be stamped with an expiration date.*

▶ *Store reagent strip bottles in a cool area.*

▶ *Do not open bottles in the presence of volatile fumes*

▶ *Do not leave lid off and expose strips to light.*

▶ *Do not touch test pads with fingers.*

▶ *Bottles opened for more than 6 months should be discarded.*

▶ *Use standardized dipstick controls on a daily basis.*

▶ *Evaluate each chemical parameter on the dipstick and record results.*

Future Trends

Dipstick urinalysis is becoming a valuable diagnostic tool. This is evident in the recent tests for microalbumin and bladder cancer detection.

The Chemstrip™ Micral Urine Test Strips (Roche Diagnostics, Indianapolis, IN) is a semi-quantitative immunochemical assay that is sensitive and specific for albumin [Hohenberger 2001]. The test detects *microalbuminuria*, the earliest sign of diabetic nephropathy (DN). Microalbuminuria is diagnostic of

Stage III DN, and is the most important factor in early recognition of the development of DN [Hohenberger 2001]. It is a stage in which further progression of the disease can potentially be stopped by a number of treatment options, including the optimization of metabolic control, lowering of blood pressure and reduction of dietary protein [Hohenberger 2001]. Elevated levels of urinary albumin proteinuria the hallmark and starting point of clinical nephropathy [Schlipdenbacher 1990]. In order to improve renal prognosis and life expectancy, DN has to be diagnosed at an earlier stage [Hasslacher 1989].

The former Bard Bladder Tumor Associated (BTA) Rapid Latex Test, is an in vitro device intended for the qualitative measurement of bladder tumor associated analytes in human urine to aid in the management of bladder cancer patients. Samples of urine from patients with a history of bladder cancer are mixed with latex particles coated with nonspecific human IgG and blocking agents. If the BTA analytes are present in urine at a significant level, they will combine with the latex particles to produce an agglutination reaction. A color change differentiates positives from negatives by use of a specially prepared test strip [Bard 1996]. Results of the BTA test should not be interpreted as absolute evidence for the presence or absence of Transitional Cell Carcinoma (TCC) of the bladder. Elevated levels may be observed in urine from patients with recent surgery, biopsy or other invasive trauma to the bladder or urinary tract. Active infections of the genitourinary tract, renal or bladder calculi, and positive leukocyte reading on urinalysis test strip may cause false-positive test results. TCC of the kidney or ureters may give a positive BTA test result. The results of the tests should be used only in conjunction with information available from the clinical evaluation of the patient and other diagnostic procedures.

References

Bard Diagnostic Sciences: *Bard BTA: A Rapid Urine Test for the Detection of Bladder-Tumor–Associated Analytes* [Package Insert], 1996.

Boehringer Mannheim Corporation: *Chemstrip™ 10 S-UA* [Package Insert]. Indianapolis, Indiana; Boehringer Mannheim, 1993.

Boehringer Mannheim Corporation: *Chemstrip™ Super UA Operator's Manual*. Indianapolis, Indiana, 1994.

Boehringer Mannheim Corporation: *Urinalysis Today*, 1991.

Bonnardeaux A, Somerville P, Kaye M. A study on the reliability of dipstick urinalysis. *Clin Nephrol* 41(3):167–172, 1994.

Brunzel NA: Fundamentals of Urine and Body Fluids Analysis. Philadelphia: Saunders, 1994.

Free AH, Free HM: *Urodynamics Concepts Relating to Urinalysis* Elkhart: Ames Company, 1974.

Harrison C: *Urinalysis With an Eye Toward Competency Assessment.* Chicago; ASCP Press, 1996.

Hasslacher CH et al: *Lab Med* 123:231–234, 1989.

Henry JB: *Clinical Diagnosis of Management by Laboratory Methods.* Philadelphia; WB Saunders, 1996.

Hohenberger EF, Kimling H: Visual urinalysis with test strips: 5. Detection of microalbuminuria with Micral-Test II. *Compendium: Urinalysis With Test Strips.* Roche Diagnostics, last updated December 2001, <demapoc.mah.roche.com/content/urinal/comp/det/det.htm>

James GP, Bee DE, Fuller JB: Accuracy and precision of urinary pH determinations using two commercially available dipsticks. *Am J Clin Pathol* 10(3):368–374, 1978.

Laux L: Visual interpretation of blood glucose test strips. *Diabetes Educator.* 1:41–44, 1994.

Miles Incorporated: *Modern Urine Chemistry Manual.* Elkhart, Indiana: Miles Incorporated, 1991.

Miles Incorporated: *Ictotest Reagent Tablets for Urinalysis* [Package Insert], 1994.

Peele JD, Gadsden RH, Crews R: Evaluation of Ames Clini-Tek. *Clin Chem* 23(12):2238–2241, 1977.

Peele JD, Gadsden RH, Crews R: Semi-automated vs visual reading of urinalysis dipsticks. *Clin Chem* 23(12):2242–2246, 1977.

Ross DL, Neely AE: *Textbook of Urinalysis and Body Fluids.* Norwalk: Appleton-Century Crofts, 1983.

Schlipdenbacher RL, Traeger U, Werner W. Recent Progress in Clinical Chemistry ??(7), 1990.

Schumann JL: *Manual of Cytodiagnostic Urinalysis* (2nd ed). Salt Lake City; University of Utah School of Medicine, 1989.

Selby JV, FitzSimmons SC, Newman JM, et al: The natural history and epidemiology of diabetic nephropathy: Implications for prevention and control. *JAMA* 263:1954–1958, 1900.

Stewart CE, Koepke JA: *Basis Quality Assurance Practices for Clinical Laboratories.* Philadelphia: JB Lippencott Company, 1987.

Strasinger, SK: *Urinalysis and Body Fluids.* Philadelphia; FA Davis Company, 1985.

White G. Twelve months' experience of a quality assessment scheme for urine tests using reagent strips. *Ann Clin Biochem* 32:589–59, 1995.

Woolhandler ??: US Preventive Services Task Force. JAMA 262(2):???, 1989.

Wet Microscopic Urinalysis

Wet microscopic urinalysis (wet urine sediment examination or wet urinoscopy) is and will remain the clinical laboratory method most commonly used to initially evaluate morphologic or formed elements (entities) in the urine sediment [Roche 1973, Bunzel 1994, Haber 1978, Henry 1996]. Carefully performed urine sediment examination following proper specimen collection is of clinical value in the early detection, diagnosis, and management of urinary infections, inflammatory conditions, intrinsic renal disorders, lower urinary tract disorders, pre-renal systemic disorders, and metabolic disorders [Henry 1996]. Urinoscopy often provides a unique biopsy-like view of the state of the renal parenchyma, tubular lumina, and epithelial cells of the upper and lower urinary tract [Haber 1978]. Accurate identification of a renal cast may be as diagnostically important as a tissue biopsy in revealing the nature of the pathologic change in the renal tubule; it not only makes available knowledge of the contents of the tubule, but offers morphologic information on the location of the urinary system lesion and the degree of distortion [Roche 1973].

We believe that a complete wet microscopic urinalysis is necessary in all patients. However, some healthcare providers recommend that microscopic examination of urinary sediment is only indicated: 1) when a patient is symptomatic; 2) when a patient has a positive history; 3) when there is abnormal urine color or appearance; 4) when there are positive dipstick urinalysis results; or 5) when requested by a physician. Each healthcare provider should determine the most appropriate and cost-effective urinalysis protocol to meet the demands of the patient population served.

In the early 1980s, standardized systems were developed for performing routine wet microscopic urinalysis. In 1986, one of us (GBS) reported that manual slide systems that were commercially available proved to be far superior to the conventional 22 × 22mm glass-slide method [Schumann 1986]. Since then, there has been increasing evidence that the conventional "1-drop" method is imprecise and should not be considered a standardized wet microscopic urinalysis method. Some investigators called for more correlative studies to determine the efficiency of manual or automated systems for standardized wet microscopic urinalysis [Henry 1996, Schumann 1986].

Automated and Semi-Automated Systems

In addition to manual standardization, wet microscopic urinalyses have become automated and semiautomated. One such automated instrument is the Yellow Iris (International Remote Imaging Systems, www.proiris.coom). No centrifugation or slide is needed to perform the microscopic analysis of the urinary sediment. Urine is poured directly from the specimen collection container into the instrument, and the formed elements are detected by a video camera. This automated system requires operator intervention—to our knowledge, a complete "walkaway" system has yet to be developed. Sysmex Corporation of America (www.sysmex.com) has recently introduced an automated system using flow cytometry. The advantages, cost-effectiveness and limitation of these systems require further studies.

Recently, two new "closed" manual and semiautomated microscopic urinalysis systems have been introduced to the clinical laboratory. The Cen-Slide™ system (Avstar, Newport Beach, CA) is an easy-to-use, safe, manual system that eliminates decanting, pipetting, and coverslipping of the microscopic slide. It consists of a flat-base slide viewing area in an unbreakable disposable unit.

The R/S 2000/2003™ system (www.diasyscorp.com) involves a "wrap around" workstation that consists of a control unit. This unit contains a peristaltic-type pump, valves, electronic circuitry, and a closed glass optical slide assembly or chamber that eliminates the use of pipettes, slides, and coverslips. The R/S 2000 and the R/S 2003 use the same patented slide assembly. The R/S 2003 is an enhanced R/S 2000 with a more powerful pump for increased peristaltic action and components for improved maintenance and cleaning.

Both manufacturers emphasize the safety benefits of not handling the sample. Also, they report comparable results with these systems and the KOVA™ (ICL Scientific, Fountain Valley, CA) microscopic urinalysis system.

Physical features of widely used standardized microscopic urinalysis systems were compared. We also evaluated the distribution of sediment elements with the five systems. The sediment volume and distribution, microscopic viewing surface, and microscopic clarity were evaluated [Schumann 1996]. Physical features and some differences of each slide system are listed in **T**5.1. We compared cellular counts in samples with low concentrations of RBCs (trace to 2+ reagent strip reactions) and with low levels of WBCs (trace to 2+ reagent strip reactions). In addition, we compared wet microscopic urinalysis findings in "known" sediments containing mucus, bacteria, fungi, casts, crystals and epithelial cells and fragments and correlated these with specialized confirmatory cytodiagnostic urinalysis. None of the systems had a problem with morphologic recognition of common sediment entities. Various

T5.1 **Physical Features of Unstandardized Conventional and Standardized Wet Routine Urinalysis Slide Systems***

Parameter	Conventional	Uri-Slide™	KOVA™	Count-10™	Cen-Slide™	R/S 2000/2003™
System type	Open	Open	Open	Open	Closed	Closed
Slide /case	1	1	1	1	1	1
Maximum cases/slide	1	4/10	4/8	10	1	NA
Slide	Glass	Plastic	Plastic	Plastic	Plastic	Glass
Coverslip	Glass	Glass	Plastic	Plastic	Plastic	NA
Grids available	No	Yes	Yes	No	No	Yes
Sediment volume (μL) Variable	50 μL	16 μL	6 μL	6 μL	30 μL	5 μL
Viewing area (mm)	484	90	32	36	88	38
No. of 100× fields (low power)	144	25	9	12	30	21
No. of 400× fields (high power)	2,116	420	119	49	432	196
No. of visual focal planes	1–2	1–2	1–2	3–4	3–4	1–2

*Uri-Slide (Fisherbrand, Pittsburgh, PA), KOVA (ICL Scientific, Fountain Valley, CA); Count-10 (V-Tech, Palm Desert, CA); Cen-Slide (Davstar California, Newport Beach, CA), R/S 2000/2003 (Diasys, Waterbury CT).

T5.2 **Comparison of Cellular Values for Five Routine Microscopic Wet Urinalysis Systems**

System	RBCs Trace to 1+ Range	Mean/Value	CV%	RBCs 2+ Range	Mean/Value	CV%	WBCs Trace to 1+ Range	Mean/Value	CV%	WBCs 2+ Range	Mean/Value	CV%
Uri-Slide™	1–2	2	0.1	8–13	11	0.9	4–6	5	0.1	22–27	11	0.9
KOVA™	0–2	1	0.1	4–10	7	1.7	2–3	3	0.1	14–18	7	1.7
Count-10™	0–1	1	0.1	1–7	4	1.0	2–5	3	0.1	12–20	4	1.0
Cen-Slide™	0–1	1	0.1	40–73	57	20.0	2–5	3	0.1	20–45	57	20.0
R/S 2000™	0–1	1	0.1	4–11	8	14	2–4	3	0.1	14–20	8	14

*Uri-Slide (Fisherbrand, Pittsburgh, PA), KOVA (ICL Scientific, Fountain Valley, CA); Count-10 (V-Tech, Palm Desert, CA); Cen-Slide (Davstar California, Newport Beach, CA), R/S 2000/2003 (Diasys, Waterbury CT).

CV, coefficient of variation.

Wet Urinalysis

sediment elements correlated acceptably with confirmatory cytodiagnostic urinalysis results. Although not required, phase contrast or supravital stain would increase morphologic detail. However, these systems cannot accurately identify epithelial alterations and neoplastic cellular changes. Detailed nuclear and cytoplasmic features are not recognizable using wet urinoscopy and require cytologic methodology [Schumann 1996, Schumann 1995].

Clinical Utility of Wet Urinoscopy

The most important clinical laboratory responsibility in the microscopic examination of urine sediment is to reliably distinguish the contents of "normal" sediment from that of "abnormal" sediment [Schumann 1996, Schumann 1995, Birsch 1994, Fogazzi 1994]. To determine whether an increase of any sediment elements is present and whether this increase indicates a pathologic condition of the urinary tract, sediment examination results need to be precise, accurate, and reproducible. Urinoscopists need to establish laboratory procedures that promote accurate recognition and diagnosis of disease states [Schumann 1996].

Hematuria and leukocyturia (pyuria) are important clinical signs of urinary tract disorders or disease. An assessment of erythrocyturia vs hematuria, pyuria or leukocyturia is often initially performed in the physician's office and the clinical laboratory. Up to three RBCs and up to two WBCs per HPF may be found in normal individuals. Persistent excretion of more than three RBCs per HPF indicates that further evaluation of the genitourinary tract is necessary. While other researchers have assessed high levels of RBCs and WBCs with these systems, our study sought to determine how the system would perform at normal or borderline abnormal level of RBCs and WBCs. When

comparing routine urinalysis results using low concentrations of RBCs and WBCs (trace to 2+ reagent strip reactions), similar enumerations were produced among systems, except lower values were observed with the Count-10™ system. Comparable results were observed with the R/S 2000™ and the KOVA™ and Uri-Slide™ systems. Manufacturers reference ranges (normals) for wet routine microscopic urinalysis are listed in **T**5.3.

Examination of known urine sediment samples containing mucus, crystals, RBCs, WBCs, bacteria, fungi, casts, and epithelial cells, by the various systems yields accurate results **T**5.4. Quantitative evaluation of the Cen-Slide is impeded by numerous focal planes and poor clarity of plastic. As with all wet microscopic urinalysis systems, further morphologic characterization of cellular casts, epithelial abnormalities, and inclusion cells is required.

In the 1970's and 1980's, clinical laboratories often were selective in deciding which urine specimens required microscopic evaluation. In 1979, the usefulness of macroscopic urinalysis as a screening procedure was proposed. A wet microscopic examination was necessary only in those patients for whom routine chemistries were macroscopically positive or in symptomatic individuals with or without known renal or urinary tract disease. Since that time, improvements have been made and the conventional method deplored as a standardized microscopic procedure.

New urine technology allows a rapid assessment of urine sediment, often in less time that the 2 minutes required for dipstick urinalysis. Further outcome studies are needed to establish the efficacy of chemical or dipstick screening protocols for wet urinalysis.

A variety of microscopic techniques for unstained urine sediment specimens have been suggested (**T**5.5). Brightfield microscopy represents the most common method used. Image contrast enhances morphologic detail, but the method has not gained acceptance in most medical institutions. Various supravital staining

T5.3 **Normal Values of Standardized Wet Routine Microscopic Urinalysis Findings***

System	RBCs/HPF	WBCs/HPF	Urinary Sediment Entities Casts/LPF	Crystals (Nonpathologic)	Bacteria
Uri-Slide™	0–3	0–8	0–2 Hyaline		
KOVA™	0–3	0–5		0–3	0–5
Count-10™					
Cen-Slide™					
R/S 2000™	0–3	0–5	0–2 Hyaline		

Each urinalysis laboratory should establish its own normal ranges based on its patient population.

*Uri-Slide (Fisherbrand, Pittsburg, PA), KOVA (ICL Scientific, Fountain Valley, CA); Count-10 (V-Tech, Palm Desert, CA); Cen-Slide (Davstar California, Newport Beach, CA), R/S 2000/2003 (Diasys, Waterbury CT).

CV, coefficient of variation.

T5.4 Comparison of Reagent-Strip Reactions and Urine Sediment Elements Findings with Four Wet Standardized Microscopic Urinalysis Systems* and Confirmatory Cytodiagnostic Urinalysis

Sample	Reagent-Strip Reaction		Uri-Slide™ (10 HPFs)	KOVA™ (10 HPF)	Count-10™ (10 HPF)	R/S 2000/2003™ (10 HPF)	Cytodiagnostic Urinalysis
1	3+ 3+ 3+	Blood Protein Esterase	>1,000 RBC >1,000 WBC	>1,000 RBC >1,000 WBC	>1,000 RBC >1,000 WBC	>1,000 RBC >1,000 WBC Mucus	Isomorphic hematuria Marked Inflammation Mucus
2	3+ 3+ 1+	Blood Protein Esterase	4–6 RBC 90–100 WBC	2–4 RBC 80–100 WBC	0–1 RBC 90–105 WBC	2–4 RBC 100–120 WBC	Isomorphic hematuria Mild inflammation
3	3+ 3+ 0	Blood Protein Esterase	25–35 RBC 0–1 WBC Calcium oxalate Epithelium	25–30 RBC 0–1 WBC Calcium oxalate Epithelium	30–35 RBC 0–1 WBC Calcium oxalate Epithelium	20–25 RBC 0–1 WBC Calcium oxalate Epithelium	Isomorphic hematuria Calcium oxalate Benign epithelium
4	2+ 2+ 0	Blood Protein Esterase	5–8 RBC 0–1 WBC Calcium oxalate Triple phosphate	8–10 RBC 0–1 WBC Calcium oxalate Triple phosphate	0–8 RBC 0–1 WBC Calcium oxalate Triple phosphate	4–8 RBC 0–1 WBC Calcium oxalate Triple phosphate	Dysmorphic hematuria Crystals Ischemic necrosis
5	2+ 2+ 1+	Blood Protein Esterase	8–12 RBC (dysmorphic) 4–6 WBC Casts/LPF: 0–1 Hyaline 0–1 Granular 0–1 RBC	5–10 RBC (dysmorphic) 2–4 WBC Casts/LPF: 0–1 Hyaline 0–1 Granular 0–1 RBC	4–6 RBC (dysmorphic) 2–4 WBC Casts/LPF: 0–1 Hyaline 0–1 Granular 0–1 RBC	10–15 RBC (dysmorphic) 3–6 WBC Casts/LPF: 0–1 Hyaline 0–1 RBC	Renal Bleeding Mucus Casts/LPF: Pathologic casts
6	Trace 3+ 2+	Blood Protein Esterase	0–1 RBC 90–105 WBC 2+ Fungi	0–1 RBC 90–105 WBC 2+ Fungi	0 RBC 90–105 WBC 2+ Fungi	0–1 RBC 95–115 WBC 2+ Fungi	Fungal UTI
7	3+ 3+ 0	Blood Protein Esterase	7–18 RBC 90–105 WBC 2–3+ Bacteria	7–15 RBC 25–35 WBC 2–3+ Bacteria	7–10 RBC 20–22 WBC 2–3+ Bacteria	6–10 RBC 20–30 WBC 2–3+ Bacteria	Bacterial UTI Reactive urothelium
8	0 3+ 0	Blood Protein Esterase	2–3 RBC 0–1 WBC Triple phosphate Calcium oxalate	1–2 RBC 0–1 WBC Triple phosphate Calcium oxalate	0–1 RBC 0–1 WBC Triple phosphate Calcium oxalate	0–1 RBC 0–1 WBC Triple phosphate Calcium oxalate	Normal Normal Triple phosphate Calcium oxalate
9	0 Trace 0	Blood Protein Esterase	0–1 RBC 0–1 WBC Uric acid	0–2 RBC 0–1 WBC Uric acid	0–2 RBC 0–1 WBC Uric acid	0–2 RBC 0–1 WBC Uric acid	Normal Normal Uric acid

10	Trace
	3+
	0
		Blood
		Protein
		Esterase
			5–10 RBC
			
			6–14 WBC
			Squamous
			Atypical
			  urothelium
				5–10 RBC
				
				8–18 WBC
				Squamous
					4–6 RBC
					
					10–15 WBC
					Squamous
						4–8 RBC
						
						5–10 WBC
						Squamous
						Atypical
						  urothelium
							Hematuria
							
							Urothelial
							  dysplasia

*Uri–Slide (Fisherbrand, Pittsburgh, PA), KOVA (ICL Scientific, Fountain Valley, CA); Count–10 (V–Tech, Palm Desert, CA); Cen–Slide (Davstar California, Newport Beach, CA), R/S 2000/2003 (Diasys, Waterbury CT).

CV, coefficient of variation; UTI, urinary tract infection.

techniques have been recommended (**T**5.6) to improve identification of urine sediment entities. Supravital staining also has not gained acceptance because it is time consuming and the morphologic detail is insufficient.

Again, an important feature of these new closed systems is their ability to allow a rapid assessment of the urinary sediment for correlation with clinical and physico-chemical findings. These new systems provide a practical and efficient method for the immediate or rapid assessment of sediment to detect and monitor microhematuria, leukocyturia, urinary tract infections, crystalluria, cylinduria, and epithelial alterations.

T5.5 Microscopic Techniques for Unstained Urine Sediment Specimens

Type of Micropic Technique	Use and Value
Brightfield	Detects cellular elements, formed elements such as casts that are difficult to characterize
Phase-Contrast	Valuable for specimens which are too thin or too transparent ie hyaline casts
Polarized Light	Valuable in revealing doubly refractile substances ie oval fat bodies
Filters	Enhances structural detail
Differential Interference	Enhances visualization of five unstained material, enables the viewer to see the geometric shapes

T5.6 Various Supravital Staining Techniques

Staining Methods	Type	Use and Value
Sudan IV Oil Red O	Wet mount	Identify oval fat bodies and fatty casts
Methylene blue	Wet mount	Non-permanent, smear must be examined before drying, good for cellular detail
Methylene blue O toluidine	Supravital	Good for cellular detail
Sternheimer-Malbin (Crystal Violet Safrin-O)	Supravital	Identify white cells and good for cellular detail.

T5.7 Wet Microscopy Entities

Cells

Hematopoietic
RBCs
Isomorphic
Dysmorphic
WBCs
Glitter
Suspect lymphocytes
Suspect histiocytes
Multinucleated giant cells

Epithelial
Squamous
Urothelial (Transitional)
Suspect Renal
Oval fat bodies
Fragments
Abnormal cells
(Suspect malignancy)

Casts

Noncellular
Hyaline
Granular
Waxy
Heme-granular
Fatty
Broad

Cellular
RBC
Suspect WBC
Suspect renal
Broad

Crystals

Amorphous urates
Uric acid
Calcium oxalate
Calcium oxalate monohydrate
Amorphous phosphates
Calcium phosphate
Monosodium urates
Triple phosphate
Amonium biurate
Calcium carbonate
Triamterene
Hippuric acid
Hemosiderin
Crystalline
Calcium hydrogen phosphate

Ampicillin
Cystine
Tyrosine
Cholesterol
Bilirubin
Leucine
Sulfonamides
Radiographic dye
Primidone
Hematin
Indigotin
Xanthine

Microbiology

Trichomonas vaginalis
Bacteria (rods and cocci)
Enterobius vermicularis
Schistosoma haematobium

Eggs (Taenia species)
Fungi
Entamoeba histolytica

Concretions and Secretions

Fibrin
Mucus
Spermatozoa
Globules
Corpora amylacea
Concretions

Artifacts

Talc
Fibers
Pollen

Laboratory Procedure

Processing procedures are extremely important in standardizing the urinalysis results.

Procedural Steps:

1. *Centrifuge 10 mL of urine for 5 minutes at 1,500 RPM (400 RCF).*

2. *Carefully remove centrifuged specimen.*

3. *Decant supernatant to the 1 mL level.*

4. *Resuspend the sediment in the remaining supernatant by gentle agitation.*

5. *Using an appropriate pipette, load the examination chamber of a standardized slide system.*

6. *Allow the urine sediment to settle for approximately 30 to 60 sec.*

7. *Proceed to examine the sediment microscopically in a systematic fashion.*

8. *Count the number of casts in at least 10 LPFs (100×), average, and report the number of casts per LPF.*

9. *Identify and count RBCs, WBCs, and renal epithelial cells using the high-power objective (400×). Count at least 10 HPFs, average and report as cells/HPF.*

10. *Comment on squamous and transitional cells, bacteria, yeast, microorganisms, and crystals and other background and report as none, trace, 1+, 2+ 3+.*

11. **T**5.7 *lists wet microscopic sediment entities. The microscopic urinalysis must be reported in quantitative terms and the power used noted. All cellular elements should be counted and recorded using high power (400×), and casts and other formed elements observed using low power (100×).Multiply by the appropriate dilution factor, if the urine was diluted during processing.*

Reporting

Formed Elements or Entities

1. **Background:** *Refers to the cellular and noncellular material. Describe as clean, slightly dirty, or dirty.*

2. *Cellularity: Refers to the general estimate of all types of cells present. Report as scant, few, moderate, or many.*

3. *Erythrocytes (RBCs): Count the number of intact RBCs in a representative field and multiply by 10 to report the value per 10 HPF. Note RBC morphology and report as isomorphic, dysmorphic, or isomorphic/dysmorphic mixed.*

4. *Leukocytes (WBCs): Count the number of cells in a representative field and multiply by 10 to report the value per 10 HPF. Note the specific gravity of the sample, because urine that is hypotonic may alter and diminish nuclear segmentation.*

5. *Epithelium: Identify as either renal, urothelial, or squamous in origin. Epithelium can be composed of single cells or fragments, Fragments are defined by the attachment of 3 or more epithelial cells. Types of epithelial fragments include squamous, urothelial, renal and glandular.*

6. *Urine Casts: Count the number of casts in 10 LPF. Identify the specific type of cast.*

7. *Crystals: Identify the specific type.*

8. *Concretions and Secretions*

9. *Microbiology*

Limitations Of Wet Urine Microscopy

The specific gravity of a specimen can affect the results of wet microscopy. At low specific gravity 1.009, RBCs and WBCs are lysed and hyaline casts are dissolved. At high osmolality, RBCs and WBCs shrink, rendering their identification difficult. Also, a high pH has been noted to lyse casts.

Low osmolality, alkalinity, and lack of refrigeration decrease the survival of WBCs. Because formed elements in the urine, including casts, disintegrate rapidly, the specimen should be analyzed as soon as possible after collection.

Quality Control And Quality Assurance

The quality of the urine sample is the major determinant of accuracy in microscopic urinalysis. The sampling procedure, the time of sampling, and the conditions of storage affect sample quality.

The correlation between the chemical and the microscopic portions of the urinalysis can detect certain

random and analytical systematic error. Factors affecting sample quality include:

1. *Urine osmolality: Indicator of lytic conditions*

2. **High numbers and percentages of squamous epithelial cells:** *Indicator of unsatisfactory collection from female patients e.g. vaginal contamination.*

3. **Contamination:** *Samples may contain artifacts that could be misinterpreted as indicating urinary tract abnormality.*

Dipstick Correlation With Wet Urinoscopy

Microscopists must be knowledgeable about the clinical relevance of urine sediment findings as well as the common chemical abnormalities associated with microscopic interpretations. The grading system for elements found in urine is outlined in **T**5.8. Correlations between dipstick results and microscopic results are described in **T**5.4.

Techniques, Interpretations, And Other Considerations

Microscopic techniques for unstained urine sediment specimen are listed in **T**5.5. The various types of supravital stains used in wet microscopy are explained in **T**5.6. Wet preparations and supravital stains require no specimen fixation. Universal stains such as Gram stain and the Papanicoloau stain require fixative or preservatives. Confirmatory stains requiring fixation are the Papanicoloau stain, and the Wright stain. The Papanicoloau stain uses an ethanol fixation and the Wright stain is air-dried and uses a methanol fixation.

T5.7 identifies various cellular components found in the sediment. **T**5.8 reviews the dominant grading system for urinary sediment findings.

T5.8 Grading System of the Common Urine Sediment Entities

Entity	Negative	Trace	1+	2+	3+	4+
RBC/HPF	0	1–3	4–6	7–30	30–50	>50
WBC/HPF	0	<5	5–20	20–30	30–50	>50
Casts/LPF	0	<1	1–5	5–10	10–30	>30
Crystal/LPF	0	<1	1–5	5–10	10–30	>30
Bacteria	0	Trace	Few	Moderate	Many	Obscuring
Fungus	0	Trace	Few	Moderate	Many	Obscuring

References

Birch DF, Fairley KF, Becker GJ, Kincaid-Smith P: *A Color Atlas of Urine Microscopy*. New York: Chapman & Hall Medical, 1994.

Bunzel NA:. *Fundamentals of Urine and Body Fluid Analysis*. Phildelphia: WB Saunders, 1994.

Fogazzi GB, Padderine P. Ponticelli C, Ritz, E: *The Urine Sediment: An Integrated View*. London: Chapman & Hall Medical, 1994.

Haber MH: *A Primer of Microscopic Urinalysis*, Fountain Valley, CA: ICL Scientific, 1978.

Henry JB: *Clinical Diagnosis and Management by Laboratory Methods*. Philadelphia, PA: WB Saunders, 1996.

Roche: *Urine Under the Microscope*. Nutley, NJ: Rocom, 1973.

Schumann GB, Friedman SK: Comparison of slide systems for microscopic urinalysis. *Lab Med* 17: 270-177, 1996.

Schumann GB, Schumann JL, Marcussen N: *Cytodiagnostic Urinalysis of Renal and Lower Urinary Tract Disorders*. New York: Igaku Shoin, 1995.

Schumann GB, Tebbs RD: Comparison of slides used for standardized routine microscopic urinalysis. *J Med Technol* 3(1);1986.

Common Urine Sediment Entities

Commonly found urine sediment entities include background elements, hematopoietic cells, epithelial cells, fragments, casts, crystals, microorganisms, concretions, and secretions. The description of each urine sediment entity answers the following questions:

1. What is the entity?
2. What is its characteristic morphology?
3. What are common differential considerations?
4. What is its clinical significance?

All of the wet urine sediment entities described are unstained, identified with brightfield microscopy and photographed with the urinoscopist in mind, using 10× or 40× magnification.

Background Elements

Mucus (F6.1)

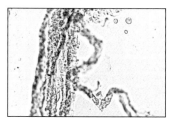

Mucus threads vary in length and are characterized by irregular length and thickness. They must be distinguished from amorphous debris, fibrin, as well as from hyaline and fibrin casts. When present in urine sediment, they are usually reported using a semi-quantitative scale of 1–4+.

Mucus is common in urine specimens containing vaginal contamination and in inflammatory conditions involving the kidney or lower urinary tract.

Fibrin (F6.2)

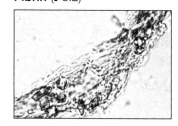

Fibrin is identified by its delicate fibrillary network and should be distinguished from the coarse threads of mucus and the cylindrical appearance of fibrin casts. Fibrinuria is reported when excessive amounts of fibrin are noted. It indicates leakage of blood coagulation products into the urinary stream. Renal thrombosis, hemorrhagic cystitis, glomerulopathies, and acute vascular rejection may produce fibrinuria. Imunoperoxidase methods are available for the identification of fibrin but are generally not required to identify fibrinuria.

Hematopoietic Cells

Urinary Erythrocytes (RBCs) (F6.3-F6.6)

Urinary erythrocytes (RBCs) are intact biconcave disks, about 7.6 μm in diameter. When observed using brightfield illumination they are a pale yellow-orange due to the hemoglobin pigment (F6.3). When the urine is hypotonic or dilute (low specific gravity), the RBCs will

F6.3 Typical urinary RBCs

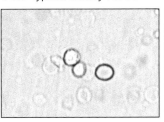

F6.4 Crenated RBCs

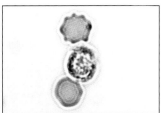

F6.5 Ghost cells

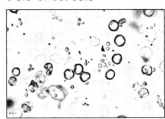

F6.6 Dysmorphic RBCs

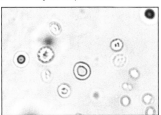

appear swollen and perfectly rounded (isomorphic). When the urine is hypertonic or concentrated (high specific gravity), the RBCs appear "crenated" and have small, evenly-distributed projections or spikes protruding from their outside membrane (**F**6.4) When the urine is dilute and alkaline, the RBCs will appear as a shadow, "hypochromatic" or "ghost" cells (remnants of cells that have burst and released most of their hemoglobin [**F**6.5]). RBCs can also be dysmorphic (**F**6.6). It is believed that dysmorphic cells indicate renal bleeding, especially from the glomerulus. They are fragmented, distorted, and contain protrusions both on the inside of the cell and the outside the red cell membrane.

The presence of RBCs in the urine is referred to as *erythrocyturia*. The presence of abnormally high numbers of RBCs in urine is termed *hematuria*.

Urinary Leukocytes (WBCs, Polymorphonuclear Neutrophils [PMNs]) (**F**6.7)

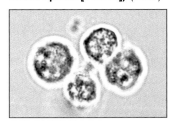

Urinary leukocytes (**F**6.7) measure approximately 10-12 μm in diameter, have two to five distinct nuclear lobes, and are about twice the size of an RBC.

The presence of abnormally high numbers of WBCs in the urine is called leukocyturia.

Urinary Epithelial Cells

Urinary epithelial cells line all of the urinary and genital tracts and unless seen in abnormal forms or numbers, represent normal sloughing off (exfoliation) of old cells. Three types of epithelial cells are commonly seen in urine and are classified according to their site of origin: squamous, urothelial (transitional), and renal.

Squamous Epithelial Cells (**F**6.8)

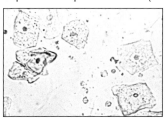

Squamous epithelial calls are large, flat cells measuring approximately 30-50 μm in diameter, with a single distinct nucleus about the size of an RBC. They are the most frequently seen and the least significant of the epithelial cells. They line the female urethra and trigone and distal portion of the male urethra.

Increased numbers are found in female urine that has not been collected using the midstream clean-catch technique.

"Clue" Squamous cells (**F**6.9)

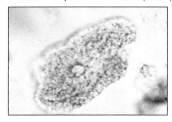

This is an especially unusual type of squamous epithelial cell of vaginal origin that can sometimes be seen in the urine. Clue cells are covered with coccobacilli, *Gardnerella vaginalis*, and indicate bacterial vaginitis caused by *Gardnerella*. The bacterium coating the squamous cell gives its cytoplasm a "shaggy" look. To be reported as a clue cell, most of the cell should be covered with the bacteria.

Urothelial (Transitional) Cells (**F**6.10)

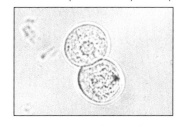

Urothelial (transitional) cells measure about 20 to 30 μm in diameter and are spherical or polyhedral. They measure about 4 to 6 times the size of an RBC. They contain a large, distinct, round or oval nucleus (roughly the size of an RBC) located centrally or slightly off center. These cells line the lumen of the urinary tract and are in direct contact with urine, which causes them to take on water, swell and vary in size.

Increased numbers of urothelial cells can be found following instrumentation. In addition, abundant urothelial cells may be found in various lower urinary tract disorders.

Renal Tubular Epithelial Cells (**F**6.11)

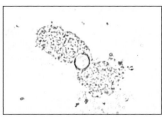

Renal cells are usually polyhedral and elongated or ovoid, with granular cytoplasm. Size will vary depending on the actual site of origin within the kidney. They are generally three to five times the size of an RBC or slightly larger to twice as large as a WBC. They will also contain a round nucleus, which is usually eccentric.

Abundant numbers of renal tubular cells are termed renalcyturia.

Urinary Epithelial Fragments (**F**6.12)

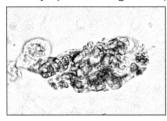

An epithelial fragment is defined as 3 or more cells that are attached to each other. The appearance of any epithelial fragment in a urinary sediment must be further investigated using confirmation with cytodiagnostic urinalysis (refer to Chapter 9 on "Indeterminates") to further distinguish urothelial from renal or glandular types.

Urinary Casts

T6.1 lists common types of urinary casts. Physiologic hyaline or granular cast should be distinguished from pathologic types.

Hyaline Cast (**F**6.13)

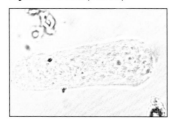

Hyaline casts are the most difficult to visualize and the least important of the casts seen in urine. They consists almost entirely of Tamm-Horsfall protein and appear as colorless, non-refractive, semi-transparent structures and can be very easily overlooked if not examined under subdued light.

Their numbers may be increased after strenuous exercise and periods of stress.

Granular Cast (**F**6.14)

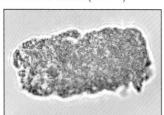

Granular casts, like hyaline casts, have little clinical significance and may be increased after strenuous exercise and periods of emotional stress. Because of their granularity, they have a slightly higher index of refraction making them easier to see. The size and numbers of

T6.1 Classification of Common Urinary (Renal) Casts

Types	Characteristic Appearance	Clinical Significance	Types
Physiologic			
Non-Cellular Hyaline **F**6.13	Transparent Cylinder	Exercise, dehydration, and fever	Nonspecific
Granular **F**6.14	Semitramsparent cylinder containing fine granules	Exercise, dehydration, and fever, accumulation of plasma proteins	Nonspecific
Pathologic			
Celluar Erythrocytic	Semitransparent or granular cylinder containing distinct erythrocyte stroma	Renal parenchymal bleeding, glomerular leakage	Glomerular disease, interstitial hemorhage (infarction)
Blood "heme" Granular **F**6.16	Red-brown granular cylinder, but intact erythrocyte stroma not seen	Same as above	Same as above
Cellular (Suspect Leukocytic)	Transparent granular or waxy cylinder containing segmented neutrophils	Renal inflammation	Tubulointerstitial inflammation (pyelonephritis), glomerular disease
Cellular (Suspect Renal Tubular Epithelial) **F**6.11	Semitransparent granular or waxy cylinder containing intact or necrotic renal tubular epithelial cells	Renal tubular damage	Renal tubular injury, acute tubular necrosis, acute allograft rejection, tubulointerstitial disease
Waxy **F**6.15	Sharply defined, highly refractile, homogenous cylinder with broken off borders and indentations	Cellular degeneration	Nonspecific
Fatty **F**6.20	Semitransparent or granular cylinder containing large highly refractile vacuoles or droplets	Lipiduria	Nephrotic syndrome
Broad **F**6.19	Width of cylinder two to six times that of other casts; waxy and granular most common types	Tubular dilation and stasis	Advanced or chronic renal disease

granules within the cast vary. They are further classified into coarsely and finely granular types, though this distinction is very subjective and is not clinically significant. The term granular cast is sufficient for reporting.

Numbers may increase after fever, strenuous exercise and periods of stress.

Waxy Casts (F6.15)

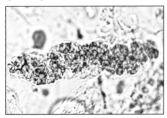

Waxy casts are easily recognized by ordinary brightfield microscopy because of their very high refractive index. They are characterized by blunt or irregular "broken-off" ends, often showing notches or indentations, or can appear smooth. They may be colorless or have a yellow-tan or pale yellow appearance. Waxy casts can often be broad and stubby rather than thin, long, and narrow.

Waxy casts indicate renal stasis and are often associated with chronic renal failure.

Red Blood Cell (RBC) Casts (Blood and Heme-granular) (F6.16)

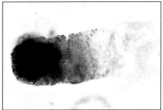

Blood casts are easily recognized due to their highly refractive nature and their color, which ranges from orange-yellow to red-brown. This characteristic color is unlike anything else seen in unstained urine sediment—impossible to miss. Blood casts are the most fragile of all the casts seen in the urine sediment. This fragility explains why we often see fragments or portions of an RBC cast in the urine. When the casts contain clearly recognizable intact RBCs in the protein matrix, we call it an erythrocytic or blood cast. As the RBCs within the cast begin to degenerate and leak out their hemoglobin into the surrounding cast matrix, the cast becomes a hemoglobin or "heme-granular" cast.

The finding of erythrocytic casts or heme-granular casts is primarily associated with glomerulonephritis. However, any condition that damages the glomerules, tubules, or renal capillaries can produce them.

Urinoscopists must be aware that sometimes blood and heme-granular casts can be "undercalled" or categorized as granular due to their lack of color.

White Blood Cell (WBC) Cast (F6.17)

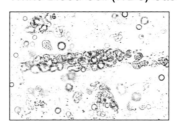

White blood cell (WBC) casts are refractile and contain easily recognizable multi-lobed leukocytes or PMNs.

They are considered pathologic and are often associated with kidney infections and differentiate upper (kidney) from lower (bladder) urinary tract infections.

Renal Tubular Epithelial Cell Cast (F6.18)

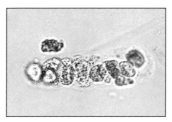

Renal tubular epithelial cell (RTCs) casts are recognized because of their high refractive index and renal epithelial cell component. Renal tubular cells lining the cast have a large eccentric nuclei, and sparse granular cytoplasm. These cells have a polyhedral elongated, or columnar shape and can either be found in rows along the length of the cast or totally embedded within the protein cast matrix.

Their presence indicates renal tubular damage or destruction.

Broad Cast (F6.19)

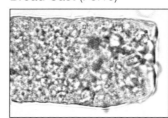

The width or diameter of a cast has become clinically significant and provides information as to the state of the tubules where the casts formed. Very narrow casts usually indicate that tubules have swollen and lumens narrowed because of an inflammatory process. Broad casts indicate a more severe pathology and are formed in dilated renal tubules or larger collecting tubules. Even though broad casts can be of any type, most are of the waxy cast type (their presence indicates urinary stasis and tubular obstruction).

Fatty Cast (F6.20)

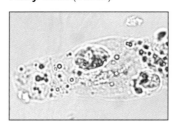

Fatty casts are easily recognized microscopically because of their high refractive index, contents of free fat or oval fat globules, and yellow-tan appearance. The lipids (fat) may vary in size and shape within the cast structure and are birefringent.

Fatty casts are pathologic and when found indicate severe renal dysfunction and is associated with nephrotic syndrome.

Urinary Microorganisms

Bacteria (**F**6.21-**F**6.22)

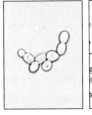

Bacteria are not normally found in urine sediment when the urine specimen is collected under sterile conditions and stored properly until it is examined. Bacteria are extremely small and can be either cocci (**F**6.21) or rod (**F**6.22) shaped in appearance. Bacteria only become significant when accompanied by large numbers of WBCs indicating a bacterial urinary tract infection.

Yeast (**F**6.23-**F**6.24)

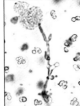

Yeast may be present in the urinary sediment as a result of contamination from the skin or air, or as a true yeast urinary tract infection. A true yeast urinary tract infection will be accompanied by large numbers of WBCs. Yeast (**F**6.23) exhibit an ovoid shape, colorless, smooth and refractile in appearance. They may also exhibit branching or hyphae (**F**6.24) with terminal buds. Yeast may be distinguished from RBCs by their smaller size (2 μm), size variability, and thick cell walls.

Parasites

Trichomonads (**F**6.25)

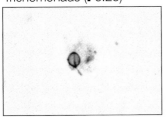

The parasite most often seen in urinary sediment examination is *Trichomonas vaginalis*. It is most commonly seen in the urine of females, but may also infect the urethra,

periurethral glands, bladder, and prostate. Trichomonads are usually searched for in wet preparations due to their distinctive rapid, very jerky, rotating movements. They are usually is pear-shaped, 30 μm long, contain a single nucleus, anterior flagella, anterior undulating membrane, and sharp protruding posterior axostyle. They are sometimes said to have an "apple-seed" appearance.

Schistosomes (**F**6.26)

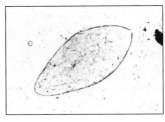

The eggs of *Schistosoma haematobium* occur in the urine; are large (from 112–170 μm long); and have a terminal spine. The parasite is found in Africa, Madagascar, Iraq, Iran, Syria, Lebanon, Turkey and India.

Enterobius vermicularis (Pinworm) (**F**6.27)

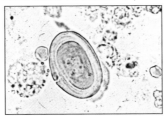

Enterobius vermicularis is commonly called pinworm, threadworm, or seatworm, and primarily infests the cecum and vermiform appendix in children. Ova are occasionally seen in the urine as a result of fecal contamination. The ova measure approximately 25 × 50 μm.

Urinary Concretions (**F**6.28)

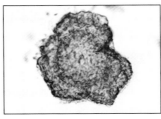

These concretions are aggregates of crystalline material characterized by fused or hobnailed-shaped structures of varied size. Their presence suggests microurolithiasis. It can be accompanied by crystals.

Urinary Crystals (**F**6.29-**F**6.37)

The presence of crystals in the urine sediment is called crystalluria. Crystals in urine can be either normal (physiologic) or abnormal (pathologic). They are further subdivided into normal acid crystals (crystals seen in normal urine of acid pH), normal alkaline crystals (crystals seen in normal urine of alkaline pH),

F6.29 Uric acid

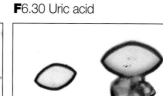

F6.30 Uric acid

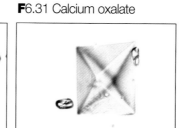

F6.31 Calcium oxalate

F6.32 Triple phosphate

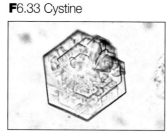

F6.33 Cystine

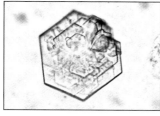

F6.34 Tyrosine

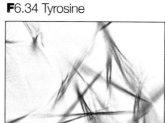

F6.35 Leucine

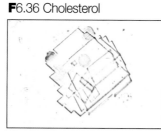

F6.36 Cholesterol

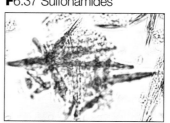

F6.37 Sulfonamides

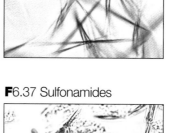

abnormal crystals of metabolic origins, and abnormal crystals of iatrogenic origin (result from medication or treatment).

Crystals are identified on the basis of morphology, urinary pH, and in some situations, solubility in heated acids or alkalies. **T**6.2 lists the common physiologic crystals encountered in the urine sediment along with their pH, color, shape, and confirmatory tests. **T**6.3 lists the abnormal crystals found in the urine sediment.

T6.2 Physiologic Crystals in the Urine Sediment: Description and Common Solubilities

Crystals	pH	Color	Shape	Heat	10% Sodium Hydroxide	Glacial Acetic Acid
Normal Acid Crystals						
Amorphous urates	Acid	Pink or red	Amorphous	Soluble at 60°C	Soluble	Changed to uric acid
Uric acid **F**6.29–6.30	Acid	Yellow or red-brown	Large variety—rhombic, rosettes, 4-sided plates, "whetstones," lemon-shaped	Soluble at 60°C	Soluble	Insoluble
Acid urates	Acid or neutral	Brown	Small spheres, clusters, resemble biurates	Soluble at 60°C	Soluble	Changed to uric acid
Monosodium urate	Acid	Colorless	Slender needles or amorphous precipitate			
Calcium oxalate **F**6.31	Acid or alkaline	Colorless	Oval, ovoid rectangle, dumbell			
Normal Alkaline Crystals						
Amorphous phosphates	Alkaline	Colorless	Amorphous granules	Insoluble		Soluble
Triple phosphate **F**6.32	Alkaline or neutral	Colorless	3 to 6-sided prisms-coffin lids, flat, fern-leaf, sheets, flakes			Soluble
Calcium phosphate	Alkaline	Colorless	Slender prisms with 1 wedgelike end, often in rosettes, flat plate	Insoluble		Soluble
Ammonium biurate	Alkaline	Dark yellow or brown	Spheres or "thorn apples"	Soluble at 60°C		Slowly change to uric acid
Calcium carbonate	Alkaline	Colorless	Tiny spheres in pairs or fours			Soluble

T6.3 Abnormal Crystals in the Urine Sediment: Description and Confirmatory Tests

Crystals	pH	Color	Shape	Confirmatory Test
Crystals of Physiologic (Metabolic) Origin				
Cystine (most common physiologic/ abnormal crystals (**F**6.33)	Acid	Colorless	Transparent, usually refractile six-sided plates. May polarize (depending on thickness	Cyanide nitroprusside reaction—red purple color
Tyrosine (rare) (**F**6.34)	Acid	Colorless (Usually appear black with focusing	Fine, silky needles arranged	Nitrosonaphthol test—orange color
Leucine (extremely rare) (**F**6.35)	Acid	Yellow	Oily appearing spheres with radical and concentric striations Usually occur with Tyrosine	Amino acid separation
Cholesterol (rare) (**F**6.36)	Acid or neutral	Colorless	Flat plate with corner notch (Seen with large proteinuria and after refrigeration)	
Bilirubin (uncommon)	Acid or neutral	Reddish brown	Amorphous needles, rhombic plates or cubes; may color uric acid crystals	
Hemosiderin	Acid or neutral	Golden brown	Granules, in clumps, in cells, casts	Blue with Prussian blue reaction (Rous test)
Crystals of Iatrogenic Origin (Drugs)				
Sulfonamides (**F**6.37)	Acid	Yellow to brown	Various—depends on the drug, mimics various forms of uric acid/urates/biurates	For all forms: Hydrolyze with heat and acid, apply diazo reaction—magenta color
Sulfadiazine	Acid	Brown	Dense globules	
Acetylsulfamethoxazole	Acid	Brown	Dense spheres or irregularly divided spheres	
Ampicillin (Penicillins)	Acid	Colorless	Long slender needles, form clusters. Sheaves after refrigeration	
Radiographic media (meglumine diatrizoate)	Acid	Colorless	Flat plates, some with corner notch like cholesterol;	Specific gravity >1.035; false-positive SSA protein test
Acyclovir	Alkaline	Colorless	Fine slender needles	Infrared analysis and/or clinical history

Note: Abnormal crystals must be confirmed by chemical test or clinical history before reporting.

Modified from Schumann GB, Schweitzer SC: *Examination of urine.* In Henry JB. ed: *Clinical diagnosis and management by laboratory methods; ed 18*. Philadelphia, 1991, WB Saunders, p 429-430.

Secretions

Corpora Amylacea (F6.38)

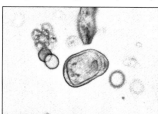

This prostatic secretion can be seen in the urine sediment of men with benign prostatic hypertrophy. Corpora amylacea are oval structures composed of a waxy, homogenous material arranged in concentric rings. Spermatozoa, prostatic ductal epithelial cells, and seminal vesicle cells are often seen in association with corpora amylacea, providing further evidence of prostatic origin. These structures should not be confused with waxy casts—corpora amylacea lack parallel sides and blunt ends and are arranged in concentric laminated rings.

Urinary Globules (F6.39)

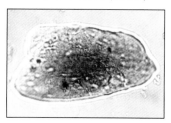

These globules are pseudocasts, and are composed of a hyaline to granular mucoprotein substance. However they lack the cylindrical shape of a renal cast and do not have the characteristic parallel sides and blunt ends typical of true casts. Urinary globules have scalloped or fluted edges, which contain small vacuoles. They may be found in the urine sediment of patients with reflux nephropathy, obstructive uropathy and urinary stasis. They represent congealed urine that has leaked from the renal tubules into the interstitial spaces of the kidneys.

Seminal Vesicle Fluid (Sperm) (F6.40)

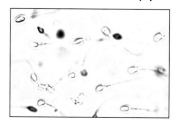

Seminal vesicle fluid consists of a combination of many products of the male reproductive organs. The product most often seen is sperm.

Normal Wet Urinalysis Findings

It is important that the clinical laboratorian distinguish wet urinalysis (physiochemical and microscopic urine sediment) results that represent *"normal"* or *"negative"* findings from *"abnormal"* findings. This chapter will provide physicians, nurses, and clinical laboratory professionals with the most current "normal" values for the commonly used wet urinalysis tests. Urinalysis laboratories need to develop their own reference values for *"normal"* urine based on their particular methodology and their patient population.

Chapter 8 describes the findings of an *"abnormal"* wet urinalysis, Chapter 9 describes the findings associated with *"indeterminate"* or *"inconclusive"* wet urinalysis results.

T7.1 Reference Values for Normal Physical and Dipstick Urinalysis Testing

Parameter	Range
Physicochemical Analysis	
Color	Yellow, deep yellow, amber
Clarity	Clear
Dipstick Urinalysis	
Specific Gravity	1.000–1.035 (Adult Random Urine)
pH	5–7
Protein	Negative–Trace (15 mg/dL)
Glucose	Negative
Ketone	Negative
Bilirubin	Negative
Blood	Negative
Nitrite	Negative
Leukocyte Esterase	Negative
Urobilinogen	≤ 1.0 mg/dL or ≤ 1 Ehrlich Unit/dL

T7.2 Reference Values (Normal) for Other Urine Chemistry Testing

Parameter	Range
Qualitative Analysis:	
Ictotest™ (Bilirubin) Test	Negative
Semi-Quantitative:	
Sulfosalicylic Acid (SSA) Test (Total Protein)	150 mg/24 hrs or 10 mg/dL (Random urine)
Clinitest™ (sugars)	Negative
Reducing substances	Negative
Microalbumin (Micral Dipstick Test)	Negative
Quantitative Analysis:	
Total Protein	0–150 mg/L (Random urine)
Microalbumin	0–38.6 mg/L (Random urine)

Physical and Chemical Examination of Urine

T7.1 lists the reference values of normal urine when examined for its physical and chemical properties, (color, clarity and dipstick chemical urinalysis). **T**7.2 lists reference values for normal urine of other non-dipstick chemistries performed. **T**7.3 lists reference values (normal) for microscopic examination of the urinary sediment.

Urine Sediment Examination

Normal urine sediment contains little to no formed elements. The appearance of small numbers of abnormal sediment entities (RBCs, WBCs, hyaline and granular casts) can be normal. When numbers exceed reference

T7.3 **Reference Values (Normal) for Urinary Sediment**

Sediment Entities	Sediment Range
Hematopoietic Cells	
RBC (Isomorphic)	0-3/HPF
WBC (Neutrophilic)	0-5/HPF
Casts	
Hyaline Casts	0-2/LPF
Granular Casts	0-2/LPF
Epithelial Cells	
Squamous	Few/LPF
Urothelial (Transitional)	Few / HPF
RTC (Renal Tubular Cells)	0-1/HPF
Microbiology	
Bacteria	None/HPF
Fungus	None/HPF
Parasites	None/HPF
Crystals	
Physiologic	None/LPF
Pathologic	None/LPF
Concretions	None/HPF
Lipids	None/HPF

LPF, Low Power Field (10× objective); HPF = High Power Field (40× objective).

values, these indicate "true" abnormal wet urinalysis findings. The individual sediment entities that comprise a normal urine will now be discussed.

Hematopoietic Cells in "Normal" Urine

This category includes any cells present in the blood (hematopoietic cells) that can also be found in the urine sediment. The most common cells are erythrocytes (RBCs) and leukocytes (WBCs), often referred to as polymorphonuclear cells (PMNs) or neutrophils.

Urinary Erythrocytes (RBCs)

The presence of a few erythrocytes (isomorphic) is considered normal or benign, and any number greater than 3 RBCs/HPF is considered abnormal and may represent an early indication of possible renal disorders or disease, trauma, infection, stone formation, or possibly a tumor.

Morphology of the urinary RBCs has aided the urinoscopist in determining the site of hematuria. The occurrence of dysmorphic (distorted, irregular) RBCs indicates bleeding of glomerular origin. Dysmorphic RBCs represent fragmentation of the cells as they pass through the glomerulus. Fragmentation is due to loss and damage of the RBC membrane, which does not allow it to maintain its isomorphic shape. Dysmorphic RBCs are associated with physiologic conditions such as stress and strenuous exercise, as well as pathologic conditions such as renal disease or glomerular damage. Isomorphic RBCs often represent bleeding or hemorrhage from capillaries,

or larger blood vessels. When hematuria consists of isomorphic (regular) RBCs, the bleeding is usually associated with the lower urogenital tract or bladder lesions. It is important to note that severe glomerular damage and tubular lesion can produce capillary bleeding, which yields isomorphic RBCs in the urine.

The determination of the course and site of hematuria requires both clinical information (history and physical examination) as well as physical, chemical, and microscopic analysis of patient urine. Keep in mind that a specimen appearing macroscopically normal may contain small but pathological numbers of RBCs microscopically. Therefore, it is to the diagnostic advantage of the clinical laboratory to perform microscopic examination of urine sediment on all urines.

Urinary Leukocytes (WBCs)

Fewer than 5 leukocytes/HPF are found in normal urine; more than this is considered abnormal. WBCs, like RBCs, may enter the urine along any point of the urinary tract, either through the glomerulus or from capillary trauma to the kidney or lower urogenital tract. The presence of increased numbers of WBCs is clinically called *pyuria* and usually indicates an infection or inflammation of the genitourinary system. Wet urinalysis laboratories use the term *leukocyturia* to indicate increased numbers of WBCs.

Epithelial Cells

It is not unusual to find a few epithelial cells in "normal" urine because of the normal sloughing off (exfoliation) of old cells that line the genitourinary tract. Three types of epithelial cells are seen in a "normal" urine: squamous, urothelial (transitional) and renal.

Squamous Epithelial Cells

Squamous epithelial cells are the most frequently encountered by the urinoscopist. The presence of a few squamous cells have really no clinical significance. The presence of numerous squamous epithelial cells usually indicates vaginal or perineal contamination in urine of females and foreskin contamination in males.

Urothelial (Transitional Epithelial) Cells

Like squamous epithelial cells, the presence of a few transitional epithelial or urothelial cells are seldom considered abnormal or pathologic. Increased numbers of urothelial cells and fragments are observed following instrumentation. When urothelial cells show abnormal

Wet Urinalysis

morphology, such as unusual arrangements or nuclear irregularities, the possibility of neoplasm should be considered.

Renal Tubular (Epithelial) Cells (RTCs)

Renal tubular cells (RTCs) are an important type of epithelial cells found in the urine. Increased numbers (>1/HPF) may result from a variety of renal disorders, especially tubular injury/damage (acute tubular necrosis), and renal transplant rejection.

Casts In "Normal" Urine

Hyaline cast

The most frequently seen of all casts is the hyaline cast, which consists almost entirely of Tamm-Horsfall protein. The presence of 0 to 2 hyaline casts per LPF is considered normal. Increased amounts have been detected in the sediment following stress, strenuous exercise and dehydration. In a normal individual, increased numbers should disappear in 24–48 hours. The hyaline cast only becomes a pathologic concern when found in large numbers or when accompanied by proteinuria. Conditions such as acute glomerulonephritis, pyelonephritis, chronic renal failure, and clinical congestive heart failure, can present in early stages with numerous hyaline casts.

Granular casts

Granular casts originate within the nephron by a process of gelation of the urinary proteins and incorporation of particulate material in the urine. The presence of 0 to 2 granular casts per LPF is considered normal. Granular casts, like hyaline casts, can appear in increased numbers following stress and strenuous exercise. They may be significant when present in increased numbers or when associated with glomerular and/or tubular disorders.

Microorganisms in "Normal" Urine

Bacteria

Bacteria is not normally present in urine, unless the specimen was collected under nonsterile conditions or is contaminated by organisms from the vagina or urethra.

When present in urine the condition is called *bacteriuria*. The absence or presence of bacteria in any given urine sediment is not nearly as important as whether or not the microorganisms are accompanied by inflammatory cells and measurable amounts of protein [Haber 1978, Ames 1978]. When bacteriuria is present in conjunction with large numbers of inflammatory cells (neutrophils), a bacteria urinary tract infection must be ruled out.

Fungi

Fungi are also not normally present in urine and if present probably result from contamination. When found in urine it is called *funguria*. The only time funguria is considered to be pathologic is when it is accompanied by large numbers of inflammatory cells. A fungal urinary tract infection must then be ruled out.

Crystals in "Normal" Urine

Urine crystals are not present in normal urine. Crystals found in urine (crystalluria) should be classified as physiologic (normal) or pathologic (abnormal). Crystalluria can be further subclassified as being acid (pH≤7) crystals or alkaline (pH≥7) crystals. It is important to distinguish physiologic crystalluria from abnormal or pathologic crystalluria. The latter includes: 1) abnormal crystalluria of metabolic origin (4+ uric acid, 4+ calcium oxalate, etc.) 2) pathologic crystalluria (tyrosine, leucine, crystine, etc) and 3) crystalluria caused by precipitation of drugs or medication in high doses (sulfonamides, ampicillin, etc.)

Only when reference values are known by both the provider and consumer of wet urinalysis testing can an accurate diagnosis and optimal clinical management of patients be rendered. When urine is properly collected, processed, and examined by skilled laboratory professionals using standardized, manual, semi-automated, and automated systems, precise, accurate, and reproducible results can be attained. Communicating the findings to the clinician will provide the direction he/she needs to provide the best health care.

References

Ames Inc. *Modern Urinalysis: A Guide to the Diagnosis of Urinary Diseases and Metabolic Disorders.* Elkhart, IN: Ames, 1978.

Haber MH: *A Primer of Microscopic Urinalysis.* Fountain Valley CA: ICL Scientific, 1978.

Values for quantitative total protein and microalbumin were obtained by studies performed at Dianon Systems, Stratford, CT.

Abnormal Wet Urinalysis Findings

The most important determination the urinalysis laboratory will be involved in is evaluating a patient's urine for its *"normality"* versus its *"abnormality"*. Ideally, normality of the urine is a feature of health and wellness to the examining physician, an indicator that the urinary tract is functioning properly and not producing elements that may be indications of disease. This chapter describes for the clinical laboratory professional what wet urinalysis findings determine an *"abnormal"* urine. Because wet urinalysis is a noninvasive, inexpensive, efficient procedure for early detection of renal and lower urinary tract disorders, its results will help establish a preliminary interpretation or diagnosis and suggest whether further testing is needed.

Physical and Chemical Examination of Urine

T8.1 lists the abnormal colors of urine and possible cause(s). Urine's appearance or clarity (turbidity) must also be evaluated. A freshly voided normal urine is usually clear or transparent and any appearance of cloudiness or turbidity is considered abnormal and warrants further investigation. **T**8.2 lists the most common causes of abnormal urine appearance. After the urinoscopist determines the urine's color and

T8.1 Abnormal Colors of Urine and Possible Cause(s)

Appearance	Possible Causes
Deep Yellow	Riboflavin; Nitrofurantoin
Amber	Bilirubin
Yellow-green	Bilirubin; Biliverdin
Blue-green	Dyes (methylene blue); Indicans; *Pseudomonas*; Chlorophyll
Yellow-orange	Food color; Carotene; Rhubarb; Sulfisoxazole; Phenazopyridine
Orange	Pyridium; Bilirubin
Pink	Hemoglobin; Myoglobin; Beet pigment
Red	Hemoglobin; Myoglobin; Food Color
Brown	Bilirubin; Hematin; Methemoglobin
Red-Brown	Hemoglobin; Myoglobin; Pyridium; Food Color
Black	Melanin; Methemoglobin; Phenols; Homogentisic Acid

T8.2 Common Causes of Abnormal Urine Appearance

Cause	Appearance	Comment
Crystals		
Urates	Pink sediment	Soluble at 60°C or in NaOH
Phosphates	Pink sediment	Soluble at 60°C or in NaOH
Calcium oxalates	Translucent sediment	Soluble in dilute HCl
Uric acid	Yellow-tinged sediment	Soluble in NaOH
Cells		
Erythrocytes	Red sediment	May be lysed in Carnoy's fixative or acetic acid
Leukocytes	White-gray sediment	
Epithelial cells	White-gray sediment	
Spermatozoa	Translucent sediment	Often thick, with mucoid buffy coat
Microorganisms		
Bacteria	Gray sediment	Foul odor
Fungi	Gray sediment	Sweet odor
Miscellaneous		
Mucus	Thick sediment	May be dissolved in mucolytic agent
X-ray contrast	Flecks may be noted	Soluble in NaOH
Lipids	Greasy sediment; oily substance may float on surface	Soluble in ether
Chyle	White sediment	Soluble in ether

T8.3 Reference Values For Abnormal Dipstick Urinalysis

Parameter	Value
Specific gravity	>1.030 (Adult random urine)
pH	Unexpected high or low value
Total protein (macroalbumin)	>15 mg/dL (Random urine)
Glucose	>40 mg/dL
Ketone	>5 mg/dL
Bilirubin	>1.0 mg/dL
Blood	>5 RBC/μL; Hemoglobin from >10 RBC/μL
Nitrite	Positive
Leukocyte esterase	>25 mg/dL (>10 WBC/uL)
Urobilinogen	>1 Ehrlich Unit/dL or >1.0 mg/dL

T8.4 Reference Values for Abnormal Urine for Nondipstick Chemistries

Chemical Parameter	Range
Sulfosalicylic Acid (SSA) Total Protein	>150 mg/24 hr or >10 mg/dL
Ictotest™ (Bilirubinuria)	Positive
Clinitest™ (Reducing Substances)	Positive
Total Protein	>150 mg/L (Random urine)
Microalbumin	>38.6 mg/L (Random urine)

clarity a complete chemical analysis by "dipstick" must be performed. **T**8.3 lists the dipstick determinations performed and what constitutes an abnormal result. **T**8.4 lists reference values for abnormal urines involving non-dipstick chemistries.

Urine Sediment Examination

The last determination performed on the urine and by far the most important is the microscopic evaluation. The individual sediment constituents that comprise an "abnormal" urine will be discussed.

Hemapoietic Cells in "Abnormal" Urine

As mentioned in the previous chapter, this category includes any cells present in the blood (hemapoietic cells) that can also be found in urine sediment. The most common cells are the erythrocytes (RBCs) and the leukocytes (WBCs), usually polymorphonuclear neutrophils (PMNs).

Urinary Erythrocytes (RBCs)

The presence of >3 RBCs/HPF is considered abnormal and should be termed *hematuria.* *Erythrocyturia* represents the presence of >3 RBCs/HPF in urine. Hematuria can be an early indicator of possible kidney (renal) or lower urinary tract (bladder) disease or dysfunction.

Increased numbers of RBCs may be present in the urinary sediment in the following conditions:

▶ *Renal disease, including glomerular disease, tubulointerstitial diseases, calculus, tumor, acute infection, tuberculosis, infarction, renal vein thrombosis, trauma (including renal biopsy), hydronephrosis, polycystic kidney, and occasionally, acute tubular necrosis and malignant nephrosclerosis;*

▶ *Lower urinary tract disease, including acute and chronic infection, calculus, tumor, and stricture;*

▶ *Extrarenal disease, including acute febrile episodes, trauma, blood dyscrasia, scurvy, acute appendicitis, salpingitis, diverticulitis, and tumors of the colon, rectum, and pelvis.*

Hematuria may also reflect toxic reactions to drugs such as sulfonamides, methicillin, salicylates, methenamine, anticoagulants and chemotherapy.

Not only is the urinoscopist responsible for the quantitation of the RBCs, but also an assessment of RBC morphology. The occurrence of dysmorphic (distorted, irregular) RBCs is abnormal and indicates bleeding originating from the glomerulus. When hematuria consists of isomorphic (regular) RBCs, the bleeding is usually associated with the lower urogenital tract or bladder. A finding of >500 RBCs/HPF is called *marked hematuria* which correlates with gross hematuria (brown, red, or pink colored urine) and is frequently associated with trauma, lithiasis, glomerulonephritis, acute infections, toxic immunologic reactions, and malignancies. When unexplained gross hematuria is encountered by the urinoscopist, a complete clinical evaluation is required, usually by a urologist. Referral of the specimen for cytodiagnostic urinalysis should be considered.

Urinary Leukocytes (WBCs)

A finding of >5 WBCs/HPF is an abnormal finding called *leukocyturia,* which indicates the presence of an inflammatory lesion and possible infection of the genitourinary system. Other frequent causes of *pyuria* (leukocyturia) are bacterial infections, including pyelonephritis, cystitis, prostatitis, and urethritis. Pyuria can also be present in nonbacterial disease, such as glomerulonephritis, interstitial nephritis and tumors. They may also be transiently increased during fevers and following strenuous exercise. The presence of many leukocytes (>50/HPF) and/or clumps of leukocytes in the sediment is strongly suggestive of acute infection. Repeatedly sterile cultures in this setting may indicate tuberculosis or lupus nephritis. Gross pyuria may reflect rupture of a renal or urinary tract abscess. When leukocyturia is accompanied by RTCs, the inflammatory process is considered to be renal in origin.

Calculous (lithiasis, stones) disease at any level may give rise to increased numbers of urinary WBCs because of either stasis-induced ascending infection or localized mucosal inflammatory response. Bladder tumors, as well as a variety of acute or chronic localized inflammatory processes may also cause leukocytes to be increased in the urine. The inflammatory process is a result of tissue destruction by pathologic processes, including cystitis, prostatitis, urethritis, and balanitis.

When inflammation is obscuring or where the WBCs are suspicious for lymphocytes, plasma cells, eosinophils or monocytes/histiocytes, the specimen should be considered an indeterminate wet urinalysis finding (see Chapter 9 "Indeterminate" Wet Urinalysis Findings) and cytodiagnostic urinalysis should be considered. *Lymphocyturia* indicates a chronic inflammatory process of more protracted duration since these cells produce certain immunoglobins. They represent a useful inflammatory cell population to follow during acute renal allograft rejection, lupus nephritis and during viral infections. Plasma cells in urine are associated with chronic infection, viral and fungal infection, and acute allograft rejection. Since patients with multiple myeloma have renal involvement in 60%–90% of cases, some investigators have found atypical plasma cells or myeloma cells a helpful finding in documenting progressive disease. It is important for the wet urinoscopist to be aware of the possible presence of lymphocytes or plasma cells and the need for using confirmatory cytodiagnostic urinalysis.

Eosinophils have been identified in urine of patients with drug hypersensitivities, interstitial nephritis, and interstitial cystitis. Also they have been reported in parasitic infections such as schistosomiasis. Special stains or cytodiagnostic urinalysis is required for accurate identification of eosinophils.

Histiocytes play a major role in certain chronic inflammatory processes delayed hypersensitivity reaction and following irradiation. Suspected histiocytes (and possible giant cells) found in urinary sediments need to be further characterized by cytodiagnostic urinalysis.

Epithelial Cells in "Abnormal" Urine

Squamous Epithelial Cells

Increased presence of squamous cells usually indicates vaginal or perineal contamination in the urine of females and males. The urinoscopist must always evaluate the shape and nuclear features of the squamous cells and any possible alterations should be referred for cytologic workup for the possibility of squamous cell carcinoma.

Urothelial (Transitional Epithelial) Cells

Like squamous cells, they are seldom pathologic. Only when hypercellularity holds on fragments in a voided urine sample or abnormal nuclear irregularities will the possibility of a neoplasm become apparent. The finding of epithelial (urothelial) fragments in urine may be of great diagnostic importance in identifying lower urinary tract disease. Epithelial fragments in urine originate from several sources. The most common and least diagnostic fragments represent epithelium derived from traumatic exfoliation during catheterization or instrumentation. At times their presence in urine leads to cytological "misdiagnosis" of low grade neoplasms. In contrast, the clinical importance of "true" exfoliated urothelial fragments found in spontaneously voided urine has been recognized as a diagnostic clue for urinary tract neoplasm and nonneoplastic disease. Even without associated cellular atypia, the presence of these urothelial fragments warrants close follow-up to rule out the possibility of a papilloma or low grade papillary transitional cell carcinoma.

Renal Tubular Epithelial Cells (RTCs)

RTCs remain one of the most clinically important of the epithelial cells found in urine. Their increased presence signify renal tubular injury or damage that can be caused by a variety of kidney disorders. Apart from the special circumstance of transplantation, increased numbers of renal tubular epithelial cells (or casts containing these cells) suggest acute tubular damage. They might, therefore, be expected in pyelonephritis and in the diuretic phase of acute tubular necrosis. They are also found in increased numbers in malignant nephrosclerosis, as well in some cases of acute glomerulonephritis accompanied by tubular damage. Ingestion of various drugs and chemicals may also cause significant tubular damage and exfoliation. Degenerated renal tubular epithelial cells are easily identified in the urine sediment following exposure to salicylate, nephrotoxic drugs or heavy metals.

Casts Found In "Abnormal" Urine

Casts are formed within the lumen of the kidney tubules (nephron). At the time of cast formation, any materials present within the tubule (such as cells, fat, bacteria, or other inclusions) are trapped within the cast matrix and may be visualized in the urine sediment. Casts are searched for and counted under low power and identified under the high power objective. **T**8.5 lists those casts found in "abnormal" urine and their clinical significance.

Microorganisms Found In "Abnormal" Urine

Bacteria

Bacteria are not normally found in properly collected urine, unless the specimen was collected under nonsterile conditions or is contaminated by organisms from the vagina or urethra. The presence of WBCs (neutrophils), leukocyte esterase, and nitrite may be seen with both lower and upper urinary tract infections (UTIs). Remember, the absence of any of these findings does not rule out an infection. Confirmation both microscopically and microbiologically must be performed in order to confirm a true UTI.

The finding of bacteria in urinary sediment is called *bacteriuria*. Their clinical significance depends upon the method of specimen collection and the time interval between collection and microscopic evaluation. The urinoscopist should be aware of the approximate time the urine specimen was collected. Bacteria in urine can only be indicative of a urinary tract infection if proper sterile techniques are used. Contamination of the urine specimen from sources external to the urinary tract represents a major pitfall in determining significant bacteriuria.

Urine with bacteria that is properly collected midstream, using a clean-catch techniques (into a sterile bottle and examined within 1 hour) should alert the clinician to seek infection somewhere in the genitourinary tract. Preferably, testing for bacteriuria should begin within 2 hours from the time of urine collection; but if this is not possible, the specimen should be refrigerated at 2–8°C immediately after collection and tested within 8 hours. Under no circumstances should a preservative be added to urine intended for bacteriologic culture tests.

The first-morning urine or urine that has incubated in the bladder for at least 4 hours represents the best specimen. Bacteria in urine are common and of little clinical significance unless accompanied by some other sediment abnormality, such as WBCs. Bacteria found in association with WBCs or leukocytic casts suggests possible acute pyelonephritis. Again, bacteria will be found in most urine specimens (despite meticulous collection technique) if urine is permitted to stand in a warm room for several hours.

The concentration of bacteria in urine generally serves to distinguish between urinary tract infection and contamination of the specimen. Detection of bacteria in

T8.5 Renal (Urinary) Casts In "Abnormal" States

Type Of Cast	Range	Clinical Significance
Hyaline	≥3/LPF	Stress; Strenuous exercise; Dehydration and fever; Nonspecific renal damage; Chronic renal diseases; Congestive heart failure
Granular degeneration;	≥3/LPF	Stress; Strenuous exercise; Dehydration and fever; Glomerular disease; Nonspecific renal damage; Cellular Tubolointerstitial disease
Erythrocytic	≥1/LPF	Glomerular disease
Blood (Heme-granular)	≥1/LPF	Severe renal inflammatory disease; Acute glomerulonephritis; Intrarenal bleeding (trauma, infarct)
Cellular (Suspect Leukocytic)	≥1/LPF	Acute tubulointerstitial disease (nephritis or pyelonephritis; Acute glomerulonephritis
Celluar (Suspect Renal Cells)	≥1/LPF	Tubulointerstitial disease; Acute tubular necrosis (ischemic necrosis); Acute allograft rejection
Waxy	≥1/LPF	Tubulointerstitial disease; Urinary stasis
Fatty	≥1/LPF	Nephrotic syndrome
Mixed cell	≥1/LPF	Active glomerulitis; Tubulointerstitial disease
Broad (renal failure cast)	≥1/LPF	Advanced renal disease
Crystal	≥1/LPF	Metabolic disorder
Bacterial	≥1/LPF	Acute pyelonephritis
Bile	≥1/LPF	Liver dysfunction with renal damage

LPF, Low Power Field (Brightfield Microscopy) 10× objective.

the sediment is a rapid means of alerting the clinician to the possibility of urinary tract infection until the more time-consuming confirmation procedures are obtained.

Bacteriuria is considered significant when laboratory findings show the presence of 100,000 (10^5) or more bacteria/mL of the urine specimen. If contamination of an otherwise sterile specimen with bacteria from external sources has occurred, the count may be as low as 10,000 (10^4) or even 1,000 (10^3) or less per ml. When the count is between 10^5 and 10^3, the possibility of an incipient urinary tract infection is suggested, and in such cases the physician may request that another clean-voided mid-stream urine specimen be obtained for repeat testing. Further discussions on bacterial counts can be found in standard textbooks on microbiology.

Significant urinary tract infections may be present in patients who have experienced no symptoms. Despite absence of symptoms, these infections are serious because they have the potential for causing severe kidney damage before the patient is aware of them. A significant *"asymptomatic bacteriuria"* can be defined with the finding of 10^5 or more bacteria/mL of urine in the absence of clinical symptoms. With the recent advent of simpler, less expensive methods for detecting and semiquantitating bacteruria, more and more physicians are finding it worthwhile to request bacteruria tests for high risk types of patients even though symptoms are absent. High risk types include pregnant patients, school children (especially girls), diabetic patients and patients with a previous history of urinary tract infections.

Types of Urinary Bacteriuria

Gram-negative bacteria of the type normally present in the large intestine are the organisms most commonly identified in urinary tract infections. Of these, *Escherichia coli*, *Proteus* species, *Klebsiella*, and *Pseudomonas aeruginosa* are found most frequently. Gram-positive organisms such as *Streptoccus faecalis* and *Staphylococcus aureus* cause infections somewhat less frequently. Rarely, *Myobacterium tuberculosis* is identified in the urine.

Fungi

Fungi are also not normally present in urine, and when found are usually the result of contamination. They are considered to be pathologic primarily when accompanied by large numbers of inflammatory cells (neutrophils), in which case a fungal urinary tract infection must be ruled out.

Fungi are a relatively common finding in urinary sediment. Yeast forms, usually *Candida* species, may often be seen in the sediment, especially in the urine of female subjects and of diabetic patients with urinary tract infection. Using unstained brightfield microscopy, they may be confused with erythrocytes. Other distinguishing characteristics are the ovoid shape, lack of color, variability in size, budding growth and failure to stain with eosin or the Sternheimer-Malbin stain. Branching mycelia (pseudohyphae) may be seen in the urine of patients with invasive renal parenchymal or bladder wall (cystitis) fungal infection. Another indication to use cytodiagnostic urinalysis is when suspicious fungal cells are identified. We have found that cytodiagnostic urinalysis is more sensitive in the accurate identification of fungi, especially when there is marked or obscuring inflammation. On numerous occasions we have seen phagocytosis of fungi by neutrophilic leukocytes.

Parasites

It is abnormal to find any parasite in the urinary sediment. The parasite most often seen in urine is *Trichomonas vaginalis*. Its presence is primarily responsible for vaginal infections, but can also infect the urethra, periurethral glands, bladder and prostate.

With the exception of *Trichomonas vaginalis*, animal parasites are rarely found in the urine sediment. Larvae, filaria or ova are rarely found. Rarely, the intestinal flaggelate *Giardia lamblia* may be seen (as a result of fecal contamination). Fresh water parasites may be found in urine specimens when the urine is collected in a container that has been washed with tap water. Other parasites occasionally seen in urine include: *Enterobious vermicularis* (pinworm) resulting from fecal contamination, *Trichuris* (whipworm) and *Schistosoma haematobium*.

Crystals (Crystalluria)

When crystals are found in the urine the condition is called *crystalluria*. Crystalluria is classified as being normal (physiologic), or abnormal (pathologic). Urinary crystals can be further subclassified as normal acid crystals (crystals seen in normal urine of acid pH), normal alkaline crystals (crystals seen in normal urine of alkaline pH), abnormal crystals of metabolic origin, and abnormal crystals caused by the precipitation of drugs used in high doses.

It is important to be able to distinguish normal crystals from crystals caused by a metabolic (physiologic) problem or drug-induced origin. Abnormal crystals of metabolic origin are a result of certain disease states or inherited metabolic conditions. These include crystals of cystine, tyrosine, leucine, cholesterol, bilirubin, and hemosiderin—all are infrequently seen.

Abnormal crystals that precipitate in the urine by medication or treatment are usually caused by an overdose of drugs or medication, eg, sulfonamides, ampicillin and radiographic contrast media. Abnormal

T8.6 Abnormal Crystals in Urine Sediment

Crystal Types	pH	Physiologic Normal	Pathologic Abnormal
Uric acid	Acid	X	
Amorphous urates	Acid	X	
Calcium oxalate	Acid/N	X	
Amorphous phosphates	Alkaline/N	X	
Calcium phosphate	Alkaline/N	X	
Triple phosphate	Alkaline	X	
Ammonium biurate	Alkaline	X	
Calcium carbonate	Alkaline	X	
Cystine	Acid		X
Cholesterol	Acid		X
Leucine	Acid/N		X
Tyrosine	Acid/N		X
Bilirubin	Acid		X
Sulfonamides	Acid/N		X
Radiographic dye	Acid		X
Ampicillin	Acid/N		X

N, neutral.

crystals must be confirmed by a chemical test or clinical history before reporting out.

Normal crystals are reported on the basis of morphology under low power objective. The clinical importance of identifying the crystals as to their type can put the doctor on alert to the possibility of the patient forming calculi (stones or lithiasis) of this composition. It is not unusual for stones to form without the presence of crystals, or crystals without stones. Refer to **T**8.6 for physiologic and abnormal crystals in urine sediment.

Concretions and Secretions

Concretions (Microurolithiasis)

A large aggregate of crystalline concretions is called microurolithiasis. Lithiasis is characterized by fused or hobnail-shaped structures of varying sizes. Lithiasis must be distinguished from crystals. The identification of these concretions surrounded by reactive urothelium suggests lower urinary tract stone formation, while nephro-lithiasis is suggested if the concretions are contained in renal epithelial fragments or casts or surrounded by reactive renal cells. Nephrolithiasis requires confirmation with cytodiagnostic urinalysis.

Corpora amylacea

These secretions are produced by the epithelium lining the prostate gland. They are found in the urine of

males and presence in urine is diagnostic of benign prostatic hypertrophy. They are often found with spermatozoa.

Globules

This structure, a type of pseudocast, is composed of a hyaline to granular mucoprotein. However, globules lack the cylindrical shape of a renal cast and does not have the characteristic parallel sides and blunt ends typical of casts. Urinary globules have scalloped or fluted edges which contain small vacuoles. These structures may be found in the urine sediment of patients with reflux nephropathy and urinary stasis. They represent congealed urine that has leaked from the renal tubules into the interstitial spaces of the kidney.

Lipiduria

The presence of fat in the urine is called lipiduria and indicates severe renal dysfunction. It is found in association with nephrotic syndrome, diabetes mellitus, lupus, and any conditions that causes severe damage of the renal tubular epithelial cells. Lipiduria may be in the form of free fat globules, fat within cells (Maltese or lipid-laden cells), or fat within casts (fatty casts).

Implications of "Abnormal" Wet Urinalysis Findings

Abnormal urine contains an increased levels of a chemical constituent or of formed elements in the urine sediment. Abnormal wet urinalysis findings may establish a preliminary diagnosis and prompt physician or nursing action regarding treatment and patient management. **T**8.7 lists the common types of abnormal urinary interpretations or diagnoses that can be reliably established from wet urinalysis.

Abnormal wet urinalysis results should be divided into *"conclusive"* or *"determinate"* or *"inconclusive"* or *"indeterminate"* findings. Conclusive or determinate results (**T**8.7) are reported directly.

Inconclusive or indeterminate findings require special attention. There is a dearth of literature regarding this concept and urine sediment findings associated with indeterminate findings. A disastrous pitfall in urinoscopy is "if I don't know what it is, I don't see it or report it." It is unfortunate that indeterminate wet urine sediment indeterminate findings fall between the cracks: important clinical laboratory information is missed and early treatment opportunities are delayed (see Chapter 9,

T8.7 Abnormal Wet Urinalysis Interpretations

Hematuria
  Gross
  Microscopic
  Dysmorphic (Renal Bleeding)

Pyuria/Leukocyturia
  Suspect tubulointerstitial inflammation (pyelonephritis)

Bacteruria
  Clue Cells—Bacterial Vaginosis
  Bacterial urinary tract infection

Funguria
  Monilia vaginitis
  Fungal urinary tract infection

Parasites
  Trichomonads
  Enterobius vermicularis (Pinworm)
  Schistosomiasis

Crystalluria
  Physiologic
  Pathologic

Cylindruria
  Physiologic
  Pathologic

Lipiduria

Concretion/Secretions
  Microurolithiasis
  Corpora amylacea
  Globules

Abnormal Epithelium

T8.8 Common Constituents of Abnormal Microscopic Urine Sediment Findings

Sediment Entity (Concentration 10:1)	Sediment Findings
Hematopoietic Cells	
Hematuria: RBCs (Isomorphic)	>3/HPF
Hematuria: RBCs (Dysmorphic especially Acanthocytes	>1/HPF
Leukocyturia	>5/HPF
Casts (Cylindruria)	
Hyaline	>2/LPF
Granular	>2/LPF
RBC (Heme)	0-1/LPF
WBC	0-1/LPF
Waxy	0-1/LPF
Fatty	0-1/LPF
Broad	0-1/LPF
Cellular	0-1/LPF
Microbiology	
Bacteria	≥1/HPF
Fungus	≥1/HPF
Parasites	≥1/HPF
Crystalluria	
Physiologic	≥1/LPF
Pathologic	≥1/LPF
Concretions/Secretions	
Corpora Amylacea	≥1/LPF
Globules	≥1/LPF
Concretions (Microlithiasis)	≥1/LPF
Lipiduria	≥1
Epithelial Cells	
Squamous	Increased numbers with nuclear atypia
Urothelial (transitional)	Increased numbers with nuclear atypia
Renal Tubular Cells (RTC)	≥1/HPF
Epithelial Fragments	
Suspicious Renal	≥1/LPF
Suspicious Urothelial	≥1/LPF

HPF, High Power Field (40x objective); LPF, Low Power Field (10x objective).

Indeterminate Wet Urinalysis Findings).

Abnormal wet urinalysis findings represent qualitative and quantitative assessments as well as morphology. Qualitative results describe the presence or absence of a parameter such as gross hematuria, dysmorphic erythrocytes indicating renal or glomerular bleeding. Quantitative results are useful in distinguishing normal from abnormal amounts of chemical constituents or formed elements. Quantitative wet urinalysis results are useful in establishing the severity or progression of a disorder or disease process. Instead of using qualitative reporting such as 1+ to 4+ for entities such as RBCs, WBCs and renal cells, enumeration of cells per HPF or milliliter is the optimal standardized method. **T**8.3 list ranges of abnormal values for dipstick urinalysis. **T**8.4 provides ranges of abnormal values for common nondipstick urine chemistry results. **T**8.8 list suggested values for abnormal urine sediment findings.

Indeterminate Wet Urinalysis Findings

In previous chapters, we discussed the importance of being able to distinguish when a patient's urine is "normal" and when it contains entities that make it "abnormal." The urinoscopist should correlate each of the formed elements encountered in the sediment with findings in the physical and chemical examination of the urine sample. The urinoscopist will, however, encounter entities in evaluation of the urine sediment that don't fall straightforwardly into either the normal or abnormal category: these are called *"indeterminates"* or *"inconclusive"* entities or findings. **T**9.1 lists common indeterminate wet microscopic urinalysis entities.

T9.1 **Common Indeterminate Wet Microscopic Urinalysis Findings**

Entities	Differential Diagnosis/Algorithm
Unexplained "gross" hematuria	Inflammatory conditions vs lithiasis vs neoplasia
Obscuring inflammation	Neutrophils
Uncharacterized inflammation: suspect lymphocytes, monocytes/histiocytes, eosinophils	Uncharacterized (suspect lymphocytes, monocytes, histiocytes, eosinophils) Suspect nephritis (questionable WBC casts vs WBC clumps)
Unexplained hypercellularity	Epithelium of unknown origin vs inflammation
Unexplained hypercellularity containing cells of epithelial origin	Squamous vs urothelial vs renal vs glandular
Unexplained hypercellularity containing epithelial fragments of unknown origin	Exclude urothelial fragment; exclude renal fragment; exclude glandular fragment; suspect abnormal fragment of unknown origin; unexplained reactive fragment (urothelial) vs renal
Unexplained hypercellularity containing abnormal mononuclear cells of unknown origin	Squamous vs urothelial vs renal
Unexplained epithelial fragments of unknown origin	Exclude urothelial fragment; exclude renal fragment; exclude glandular fragment; suspect abnormal fragment of unknown origin; unexplained reactive fragment (urothelial) vs squamous vs renal
Unexplained mononuclear cells of unknown origin	Squamous vs urothelial vs renal
Unexplained reactive epithelium	Squamous vs urothelial vs renal
Unidentifiable pathologic casts, both cellular and noncellular	Cellular: WBC, renal Noncellular: Suspect fatty; suspect crystalline; suspect heme-granular
Suspect nephrotic syndrome	Marked proteinuria Lipiduria: noncellular lipid; suspect fatty casts; lipid-laden cells

61

Indeterminate wet microscopic urinalysis findings are always considered "abnormalities," in that they are not constituents of normal urine, but their presence does not necessarily constitute an "abnormal urine." Importantly, indeterminate findings always require further analysis. Indeterminate microscopic urinalysis findings are by far the greatest challenge faced by the urinoscopist. The successful recognition and handling of these indeterminate entities can only enhance a patient's evaluation, add to a more accurate urinalysis result, and aid the clinician in determining whether further testing must be done to ensure his/her patient's healthcare problem is properly addressed. Comparison of normal vs abnormal urine sediment entities are shown in **T**9.2. Clinical entities and the implications of the various possible outcomes of wet microscopic urinalysis (normal, abnormal determinate, abnormal indeterminate) are shown in **T**9.3

We recommend that confirmatory *"cytodiagnostic urinalysis"* be performed on any urine sediment that contains these morphologic abnormalities. Cytodiagnostic urinalysis will further characterize indeterminate entities by assessing greater quantities of sediment, using improved cell recovery methods, and producing a permanent-stained slide of the urine sediment that can be more accurately interpreted by the urinoscopist.

Approaches to "Indeterminate" Urine Sediment Entities

The approach diagrams herein will help guide the urinoscopist in handling indeterminate entities. **F**9.1 provides a differential to the microscopic approach of a urine sediment that contains extensive hypercellularity and also appears to contain cells of epithelial origin. Cytodiagnostic urinalysis will help identify the type of epithelium present in the sediment. Cells can be morphologically classified as squamous, urothelial, renal or glandular.

The problem of unexplained epithelial fragments is demonstrated in **F**9.2. When a fragment is detected in a urine sediment, it is important that the origin and the identity of the fragment be determined. It is not considered normal for any patient to be exfoliating (shedding) fragments in their urine, unless a procedure involving instrumentation (catheterization, cystoscopy, bladder wash, etc) was performed prior to submitting a specimen. The urinoscopist must determine, according to established criteria, whether the fragment present is urothelial, glandular, or renal.

The fragments of greatest concern are those that show nuclear irregularities. These morphologic changes

T9.2 **Comparison of Normal and Abnormal Urine Sediment Entities**

Sediment Entities	Normal	Abnormal
Hematopoietic Elements		
Isomorphic Erythrocytes	0-3/HPF	>3/HPF
Dysmorphic Erythrocytes	None	>1/HPF
Leukocytes	0-5/HPF	>5/HPF
Epithelial Elements		
Squamous	Few/LPF	Increased amount; Nuclear atypia
Urothelial	Few/LPF	Increased amount; Nuclear atypia
Renal Tubular (RTCs)	0–1/HPF	>1/HPF
Fragments		
Suspicious Urothelial	None	Present
Suspicious Renal	None	Present
Microbiology		
Bacteria	None	Present
Fungus	None	Present
Parasites	None	Present
Casts (Cylindruria)		
Physiologic		
Hyaline	0–2/LPF	>2/LPF
Granular	0–2/LPF	>2/LPF
Pathologic		
RBC(Heme)	None	Present
Cellular (WBC or RTC)	None	Present
Waxy	None	Present
Fatty	None	Present
Broad	None	Present
Crystals (Crystalluria)		
Physiologic	None	Present
Pathologic	None	Present
Secretions/Concretions/Lipids		
Corpora Amylacea	None	Present
Globules	None	Present
Concretions	None	Present
Lipiduria	None	Present

HPF, High Power Field (400× objective); LPF, Low Power Field (100× objective).

F9.1 **Unexplained Epithelial Hypercellularity**

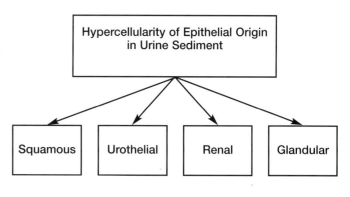

signal a possibility of a neoplasm and must be brought to the attention of the clinician for immediate follow-up.

T9.3 **Conditions, Interpretations and Implications of Normal, Abnormal Determinate and Abnormal Indeterminate Wet Microscopic Urinalysis Findings**

Clinical Conditions	Normal	Abnormal Determinate	Abnormal Indeterminate	Clinical Implications
Erythrocyturia	0–3 (Isomorphic)/HPF			Normal
Microhematuria		Dysmorphic RBCs Isomorphic RBCs		Glomerular bleeding Lower urinary tract bleeding
Hematuria		Isomorphic RBCs and blood casts Isomorphic RBCs and RTCs		Glomerulopathy; tubular injury/damage Tubular injury/damage
Gross hematuria		Explained hematuria	Unexplained hematuria	Hemorrhage Hemorrhage; neoplasm
Leukocyturia	0–5 WBCs/HPF			Inflammation; chronic vs acute inflammation; Inflammatory lesion
		Increased WBCs		Inflammation; Inflammatory lesion
Bacteriuria and leukocyturia		Bacterial UTI		Treatable bacterial UTI
Funguria and leukocyturia		Fungal UTI		Treatable fungal UTI
Renalcyturia	0–1 Renal cells/HPF			Normal
		RTCs		Suspect renal injury/damage
Fragments		Benign urothelial fragments		Instrumentation
			Suspect Renal Suspect abnormal urothelium	Suspect renal injury/damage Suspect neoplasm
Epithelial abnormalities			Hypercellularity Abnormal single cells	Neoplasm Neoplasm
Cylinduria (casts)	0–2 Hyaline/LPF			Normal
		Increased hyaline		Dehydration, congestive heart failure; stress, Strenuous exercise
	0–2 Granular/LPF			Normal
		Increased granular		Dehydration; stress; Strenuous exercise
		Heme-granular (blood)		Renal damage; Glomerulopathy
		Waxy		Chronic renal failure
		Broad		Chronic renal failure
		Cellular (WBCs or RTCs)		Tubulointerstitial inflammation or tubular injury/damage
		WBCs		Tubulointerstitial inflammation
		Fatty		Nephrotic syndrome
Physiologic crystalluria		Calcium oxalate/monohydrate		Metabolic disorder and/or possible stone former
		Uric acid		Metabolic disorder and/or possible stone former
		Triple phosphate		Metabolic disorder and/or possible stone former
Pathologic crystalluria		Cystine Lysine Tyrosine Cholesterol		Cystinuria Liver disorder Liver disorder Metabolic disorder
Urinary secretions		Corpora amylacea		Benign prostatic hypertrophy
		Globules		Obstructive uropathy
Lipiduria		Oval fat bodies		Nephrotic syndrome
Urinary concretions		Concretions		Microurolithiasis

F9.2 Unexplained Epithelial Fragments of Unknown Origin

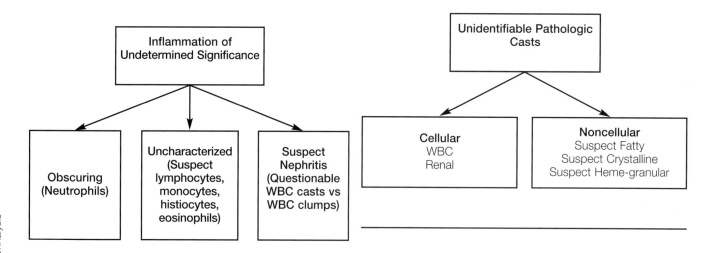

Unexplained Epithelial Fragments

- Exclude Urothelial Fragment
- Exclude Renal Fragment
- Exclude Glandular Fragment
- Suspect Abnormal Fragment of Unknown Origin
- Unexplained Reactive Fragment (Squamous vs Urothelial vs Renal)

F9.3 Inflammation of Undetermined Significance

Inflammation of Undetermined Significance

- Obscuring (Neutrophils)
- Uncharacterized (Suspect lymphocytes, monocytes, histiocytes, eosinophils)
- Suspect Nephritis (Questionable WBC casts vs WBC clumps)

F9.5 Unidentifiable Cellular and Noncellular Pathologic Casts

Unidentifiable Pathologic Casts

- Cellular
  WBC
  Renal
- Noncellular
  Suspect Fatty
  Suspect Crystalline
  Suspect Heme-granular

F9.4 Single Epithelial Cell Abnormalities

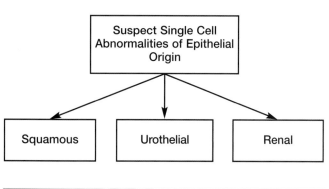

Suspect Single Cell Abnormalities of Epithelial Origin

- Squamous
- Urothelial
- Renal

F9.3 describes those situations where the urine sediment reveals severe inflammation that is either *obscuring* or simply *uncharacterized*. The urinoscopist must determine whether there are any other entities hidden under the inflammation and whether the inflammation contains neutrophils, eosinophils, lymphocytes, plasma cells, monocytes/histiocytes, or macrophages. Cytodiagnostic urinalysis can distinguish the various types of WBCs causing the inflammation. When the patient's inflammation presents as either clumps or casts, confirmation using cytodiagnostic urinalysis aids in the interpretation. Location of the inflammatory process is an important part of the microscopic examination. Presence of WBC casts indicates tubulointerstitial disease

F9.6 Suspect Nephrotic Syndrome

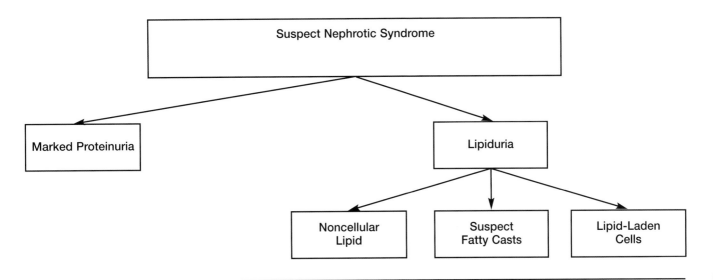

F9.7 Unexplained Gross Hematuria

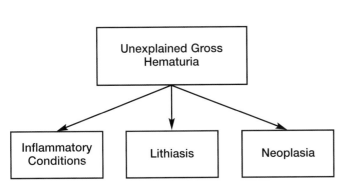

Unidentifiable pathologic casts are addressed in **F**9.5. Cytodiagnostic urinalysis is the gold standard for identifying the origin of such casts and diagnosing the underlying disease.

When suspected nephrotic syndrome is considered, it is important to document the presence of marked proteinuria and to characterize the type of lipiduria. Lipiduria can present as free lipid substances, lipid-laden cells, or pathologic fatty casts. Cytodiagnostic urinalysis, again, is the most sensitive way to identify lipid-laden cells and fatty casts. (**F**9.6)

Unexplained gross hematuria is usually associated with a nontraumatic event or injury. Gross hematuria may result from inflammatory conditions, lithiasis, or neoplasia (**F**9.7). For this reason urologic studies should be included in the early clinical workup of gross hematuria.

(nephritis) or an ascending infection. Clumps of WBCs will usually suggest bladder or lower urinary tract disease.

Sediments that present a suspicious single mononuclear cell of epithelial origin with nuclear irregularities (nuclear atypia) must not be overlooked **F**9.4. They may be the first indication of a malignancy. Determining whether the cell type is squamous or urothelial will further aid the clinician in the search for a possible location of the malignancy. The urinoscopist must also determine whether a mononuclear cell is pathologic or simply benign and reactive.

Conclusion

The urinoscopist must understand the limitations of unstained sediment analysis and the situations that require further confirmation. Indeterminate entities must be recognized and brought to the attention of the requesting clinician and pathologist or laboratory director so further testing can be initiated and the appropriate clinical management of the patient insured.

Quality Control and Quality Assurance Guidelines for the Wet Urinalysis Laboratory

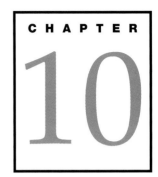

Quality control (QC) programs for wet urinalysis testing should do the following: 1) lead to decisions regarding the reliability of laboratory data, and 2) relate to the medical purposes for which the analyses are performed [Schweitzer 1986, Fuller 2001, Tetrault 2001, Travers 2002, College of American Pathologists 1984, Schumann 1984, Strasinger 1985].

A successful quality assurance (QA) program in wet urinalysis encompasses the production of results that are reproducible and precise, and from which the technologist can achieve a certain level of professional satisfaction and pride. In order to accomplish this, a QC program for urinalysis requires monitoring and regulation of steps both inside and outside the laboratory.

While most areas of the clinical laboratory have comprehensive QC systems, wet routine urinalysis has traditionally lacked the sophistication seen in other areas of laboratory testing. While discussions of QC are presented in standard urinalysis textbooks, few sources provide specific recommendations for all aspects of urinalysis testing, including specimen collection and handling, equipment maintenance, physical, chemical

T10.1 Content Requirements for Laboratory Manual

- Statement on importance of proper urine collection
- Description of type of urine to be collected
- Detailed description of specimen collection
- Specimen labeling requirements
- Delivery instructions with notations about specimen preservation
- Name and phone number of laboratory contact person for questions or problems

and microscopic analysis, ethical behavior, and continuing education. This chapter describes guidelines for a QA program for the wet urinalysis laboratory.

Quality Control and Assurance Guidelines

Laboratory Manual for Wet Urinalysis

Whether wet urinalysis is performed in the physician's office, acute diagnostic centers, or a large clinical reference laboratory, the importance of a comprehensive, up-to-date laboratory procedure manual cannot be overemphasized. The urinalysis laboratory manual should not consist entirely of manufacturers' inserts for technical and procedure information. Instead, such literature should complement written procedures, which reflect the actual materials and methods used in the individual laboratory. The procedure manual must be complete, reviewed annually, and have each review and revision signed and dated by the supervisor or laboratory director.

A well-written procedure manual provides a reference source for the bench technologist and is a tool for the instruction of nonlaboratory personnel. Supervisors, backed by specific policies that have been reviewed and approved, may also use the procedure manual for job performance evaluations or disciplinary actions. The manual must also be presented to appropriate agencies inspecting the laboratory for accreditation. **T**10.1 provides a list of minimum content requirements for a wet urinalysis laboratory procedure manual.

T10.2 Recommendations for Content of Patient and Nursing Instructions

- Statement on importance of proper urine collection
- Description of type of urine to be collected
- Detailed description of specimen collection
- Specimen labeling requirements
- Delivery instructions with notations about specimen preservation
- Name and phone number of laboratory contact person for questions or problems

Specimen Collection and Acceptability

Controlling the quality of urine specimen collection represents a major challenge, since virtually all specimens submitted for urinalysis are obtained outside the laboratory. The wet urinalysis laboratory must motivate the patient, the physician, and the nursing staff to collect a specimen that represents the true and current clinical status of the patient. Instructions for specimen collection should be written in simple language, using step-by-step illustrations. Instructions for the collection of timed specimen and special urine tests should be provided. Many patients, particularly children and the elderly, may require physical assistance in the collection of urine specimens. T10.2 summarizes important points that must be included in the instructions given to patients and nursing staff.

Following collection of an adequate specimen, the individual who accepts the specimen into the laboratory represents the first line of defense against inaccurate urinalysis results. It is to the laboratory's advantage to have written guidelines for the acceptance and rejection of specimens, and the technologist must be given the authority to implement these guidelines. T10.3 identifies criteria that can be used to reject "unsuitable" specimens. While this process of specimen monitoring is often perceived to be an uphill battle, diligence, cooperation, and communication on the part of the laboratory usually meets with success as consumers gain an understanding of and respect for laboratory standards.

Proper labeling of urine specimen containers and laboratory test requisition is the second line of defense against an inaccurate urinalysis report. The absolute

T10.3 Criteria for Rejection of "Unsuitable" Specimens

- Visible signs of contamination
- Submission of inappropriate specimen type
- Use of wrong preservative
- Incorrect labeling of specimen or requisition
- Transportation delay of specimen to laboratory (over 60 minutes, unrefrigerated)
- History not included on requisition

T10.4 Policy for Handling "Mislabeled" Specimens

- Do **NOT** assume any information about the specimen or patient
- Do **NOT** relabel an incorrectly labeled specimen
- Do **NOT** discard the specimen until investigation is complete
- Leave specimen **EXACTLY** as it was received: put in the refrigerator for preservation until errors can be resolved
- Notify floor, nursing station, doctor's office, etc, of problem and why it must be corrected for analysis to continue
- Identify problem on specimen requisition with date, time, and your initials
- Make person responsible for specimen collection participate in solution of problem(s)
- Document any action taken on the requisition slip
- Report all mislabeled specimens to the quality assurance board

minimum that should appear on the specimen label includes the patient's complete name, the date, and time of collection. Failure to meet these three basic requirements should result in rejection of the specimen. The requisition accompanying each specimen should contain the following: the patient's complete name, date, test requested, type of specimen, physician's name, and a brief, pertinent clinical history. Failure to provide this information does not necessitate rejection of the specimen, but a telephone call may be needed to complete the requirements. In the authors experience, the most common labeling error involves the mis-matching of specimens to requisition (ie, Robert Jones' urine and Ronald James' requisition). A written policy, such as the one suggested in T10.4 should be established which delineates the action to be taken within the laboratory when labeling errors occur.

Maintenance and Quality Control of Equipment

The equipment found in the urinalysis laboratory requires routine preventive maintenance. The laboratory procedure manual should include detailed, written procedures for the monitoring and care of refrigerators, freezers, centrifuges, refractometers, waterbaths, microscopes, semiautomated and automated analyzers and workstations. Service and repair records, troubleshooting guidelines, and "out-of-control" procedures should be readily available. T10.5 lists recommendations for maintenance and monitoring intervals of the equipment previously mentioned [College of American Pathologists 1984].

Several models of semi-automated and automated reagent-strip readers are available. A major advantage of these instruments is the improved reproducibility in the interpretation of the color reactions of the test strips. Manufacturers provide control solutions and reference strips for their calibration.

T10.5 **Recommendations for Maintenance of Wet Urinalysis Laboratory Equipment**

Instrument	Suggested Interval	Type of Calibration	Acceptable Range
Refrigerator	Daily	Temperature check	7 to 60°C
Freezer	Daily	Temperature check	−20°C
Refractometer	Daily	Distilled H_2O NaCl (5%) Sucrose (9%)	1.000 1.022 +/− 0.001 1.034 +/− 0.001
Urinometer	Daily	Distilled H_2O NaCl (5%) Sucrose (9%)	1.000 1.022 +/− 0.001 1.034 +/− 0.001
Water bath	Daily	Temperature check	As required
Centrifuge	Monthly	RPM and timer check	Per specifications
Microscopes	Daily Semi-annually	Kohler illumination Cleaning, repair as required	Per manufacturer Per manufacturer
Urine Chemistry Analyzers	Daily	Cleaning, repair as required	Per manufacturer
Urine Workstation	Daily	Cleaning, repair as required	Per manufacturer

Physical Examination of Urine

The physical examination of urine includes the assessment of color, clarity (appearance, character or turbidity), and specific gravity. The wet urinalysis laboratory procedure manual should include detailed instructions for the performance of this portion of the urinalysis. QC efforts in the physical examination of urine should concentrate on reducing ambiguity, improving consistency, and adopting standardized terminology to be used by all personnel. For example, the term "straw" should be replaced with the color "light yellow." The term "bloody" should not be used because it interprets red urine as hematuria, and thereby implies a particular diagnosis that cannot be confirmed prior to chemical and microscopic examination. Descriptors for clarity should comprise a small set of well-defined terms such as those found in **T**10.6.

Specific gravity determination is an important part of the wet urinalysis that should not be overlooked or omitted. Daily controls of urinometers or refractometers should consist of a zero check (distilled water) and at least one function check (NaCl or sucrose solution) [Schumann 1984a].

Chemical Examination of Urine

Chemical reagent-strip testing is perhaps the easiest component of the urinalysis to QC thanks to the availability of commercial control products. While reagent-strips represent state-of-the-art technology, their simplicity and ease of use often lead to abuse. **T**10.7 provides a list of recommendations for the proper performance of the reagent-strip test [Strasinger 1985].

QC testing of reagent-strips should be performed on every open container used by every shift. A control product should test every parameter of the reagent-strip and the limitations of the control product must be known. For example, a urobilinogen control based on an Erhlich's-positive compound will not serve as a positive

control for the BMC reagent-strip [BMC/Biodynamics 1986]. Another example is the control for leukocyte esterase activity. Because most esterase controls do not use purely human leukocyte esterases and therefore have different reactivities, these controls may not be a true representation of leukocyte activity. Commercial products available for QC of reagent-strips are convenient, but more expensive than "home-made" controls. Laboratories can also make control solutions, but this requires an initial investment of time and care in order to design a good composite control.

T10.6 **Guidelines for the Interpretation of Specimen Clarity** (Appearance or Turbidity)

Term	Definition
Clear	No visible particulate matter present
Hazy	Some visible particulate matter present: newsprint is not distorted or obscured when viewed through the urine
Cloudy	Newsprint can be seen through the urine but letters are distorted or blurry
Turbid	Newsprint cannot be seen through the urine

T10.7 **Recommendations for Dipstick Urinalysis Testing**

- Test the urine as soon as possible after receipt (30–60) minutes
- Test a well-mixed unspun urine
- Test a urine that is at room temperature
- Dip reagent-strip into urine *briefly*—no longer than one second
- Drain off excess urine—run edge of strip along rim of tube, tap edge on absorbent paper
- Do not allow reagents to run together
- Follow exact timing recommendations for each chemical test
- Know sources of error, sensitivity and specificity of each test on the reagent strip
- Make correlations between patient history and individual tests
- Keep reagent-strip container stoppered and strips properly stored

Procedural Factors
Volume of urine examined (10, 12, 15 mL)
Speed of centrifugation (400× g, 600× g)
Length of centrifugation (10 minutes)
Concentration of sediment (10:1, 12:1, 15:1)
Volume of sediment examined

Reporting Factors
Each laboratory should publish its own normal values (based on system used and patient population)
All personnel must use same terminology
All personnel must report results in standard format
All abnormal results should be flagged for easy reference

- Unsatisfactory specimen due to squamous contamination, obscuring crystals, bacterial overgrowth, etc
- Significant hematuria (specify: >50 RBCs/HPF)
- Physiologic casts (specify: hyaline) present
- Suspected pathologic casts (specify: cellular, waxy) present
- No oval fat bodies identified (answer to clinical qualitative question)
- Unidentified cells/casts/tissue fragments present; recommend confirmatory urinalysis such as cytodiagnostic urinalysis
- Suspect renal tubular injury and casts present; recommend confirmatory urinalysis such as cytodiagnostic urinalysis

Tablets, chemicals and reagent-strips should be examined before each use for visible signs of contamination or spoilage, incorrect storage, and outdate. Tablets, such as the Acetest™ and Ictotest™, should have both positive and negative controls run daily or whenever the test is used. Pediatric chemistry controls make an excellent positive control for the Ictotest™, and acetone will give a positive reaction with the Acetest™. Distilled water can serve as a negative control for both. Controls for the SSA protein procedure may be purchased or made. Care should be taken to make sure the control value is within the critical range for that particular test.

Wet Urine Microscopy (Microscopic Urinalysis)

QC of microscopic urinalysis centers on standardization of technique and adherence to details in procedure and reporting policies. The establishment of strict procedural guidelines can ensure that the same equipment is used by all personnel, in proper sequence, following the same techniques. **T**10.8 lists procedural and reporting factors for the microscopic urinalysis that must be considered, if the microscopic urinalysis is to be standardized. Throughout this portion of the urinalysis, consistency must be the primary objective, for it is here that diagnostic information can be overlooked or underestimated due to variability, subjectivity, and individuality in technique. Supervisors, backed by written standard operating procedures that are periodically reviewed and updated, should strive to encourage their personnel to improve their microscopic skills and clinical correlative ability.

Several standardized urinalysis systems are available that represent a vast improvement in the way microscopic urinalysis is performed (see Chapter 4). The manual, semi-automated and automated urinalysis systems seek to control the urine sediment, thereby standardizing the microscopic component of the urinalysis [Ross 1983, ICL Scientific 1982, Whale Scientific 1982, V-Tech 1983, Schumann 1986]. Each system includes a

specially designed slide that holds a predetermined, consistent volume of sediment and has distinct characteristics with regards to focal planes, settling times, and optical quality. Laboratories must consider these characteristics when choosing a slide system. However all are considered superior to the conventional glass slide and coverslip technique [Schumann 1986].

The use of daily controls for microscopic urinalysis is strongly recommended. However, there is no commercial control product available that adequately represents all components of the microscopic examination, particularly cells and casts. The authors recommend that the supervisor or an appointed individual select a urine sediment to be microscopically examined by personnel on all shifts. This specimen may be inserted into the work flow as a known or unknown and may then be used as the basis for continuing education activities, such as an in-lab seminar or conference.

Standardizing terminology and format is an essential component in the effective communication of urinalysis results. **T**10.9 provides examples of descriptive reporting statements that lend in-depth information. Computerized reporting is efficient and is used in clinical laboratories of all sizes, but it can be too restrictive. The technologist should not be limited to reporting "epithelial cells" or "casts," but must identify and report specific types whenever possible.

The format used to report urinalysis results should be quantitative. Many laboratories have already begun to move away from qualitative reporting (ie, 0–4+) when enumerating RBCs and WBCs. Controlling the use of ranges (ie, 5–10 WBCs/HPF) and using pre-approved terms for cellular and noncellular entities will standardize results and make flagging abnormal specimens easier. Both ranges and terms should be posted in the microscopic work area for easy reference and periodically published in laboratory communications so that clinicians may become familiar with them.

The laboratory can cross-check or verify urinalysis results through the comparison of patient history, macroscopic results, and microscopic findings. For

Wet Urinalysis

T10.10 Suggested Wet Urinalysis Quality Control Schedule

Area Checked	Daily	Weekly	Monthly	Semi-annually or annually	As necessary
Reagents and Supplies					
Reagent strip	X				
Reagent tablets	X				
Remaking protein standard				X	
Equipment					
Refrigerator temperature	X				
Freezer temperature	X				
Daily refractometer calibration	X				
Daily urinometer calibration	X				
Daily spectrophotometer calibration	X				
Microscope maintenance				X	
Thermometers		X			
Glassware			X		
Centrifuge maintenance				X	
Education					
Revise laboratory manual				X	
Technologist proficiency testing			X		
Update library				X	
Clinicopathologic correlations					X

example, if significant numbers of RBCs are identified on the microscopic examination, but the reagent-strip result for blood is negative, the specimen should be rechecked or other possible sources of error investigated. The reporting of oval fat bodies in the absence of significant proteinuria, by both dipstick and SSA testing, should alert the technologist to perform a confirmatory stain procedure for lipids before reporting such clinically important results. A pathologist should be available to review all urinalysis results with critical medical significance.

In-House Controls and External Proficiency Testing

Daily in-house controls are an excellent means of monitoring the precision and reproducibility of the work of personnel performing the urinalysis [Schumann 1986]. Every control specimen should be of sufficient volume, and should be properly stored and tested by each shift. Hidden controls slipped into the routine workload by the supervisor will ensure that control specimens are not receiving any type of preferential treatment. T10.10 lists a suggested QC schedule for wet urinalysis.

In-house controls, especially hidden controls, may be poorly received by laboratory personnel, if viewed as a threat rather than a learning experience. QC should not hurt morale, but an effective program should not be abandoned simply because the personnel do not like it. Communication and education are essential components of an effective QC program. Several recommendations to improve the way a quality control program is perceived by employees include actively involving the person(s) whose work is being monitored, emphasizing that duplicate testing allows problems to be pinpointed that may be procedural and not technologist related, and documenting the positive performance of the tech-

nologist [Stewart 1985].

Proficiency testing programs in urinalysis provide an index of the quality of interlaboratory testing and intralaboratory peer review performance. Any proficiency testing program requires active review by a pathologist or laboratory director and documentation of corrective action taken in deficient areas [Stewart 1985].

Ethical Behavior and Professionalism

All persons involved in laboratory testing must display a high degree of ethical behavior where QC is concerned. This means performing tests on controls before actual patient testing is done, recording the results that are obtained, not those one should get and taking appropriate action when controls are "out" (ie, not within the acceptable limits). Documenting any action taken to correct errors, refraining from the release of any results when problems arise, and keeping the supervisor informed about any detected problems ensure that ethical standards are maintained. The flow chart in T10.11 outlines a control procedure and recommendations for action when controls are not within the acceptable limits.

Continuing Education and Postgraduate Training

Increasing attention has been paid to upgrading the entire urinalysis procedure. Specialized urinalysis, such as cytodiagnostic urinalysis, targeted at the symptomatic patient has been developed and advocated [Clark 1985, Schumann 1984b, Schumann 1985, Schumann 1983]. Laboratories must continually work to upgrade staff knowledge and abilities, so that the quality of the urinalysis service keeps pace with other areas of laboratory testing.

T10.11 Out-of-Control Wet Urinalysis Procedures

Record all actions taken and the resolution of any problems
Use the flow diagram below:

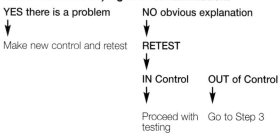

Step 1. **Run control**

IN Control   OUT of Control

↓   ↓

Proceed with testing   Go to Step 2

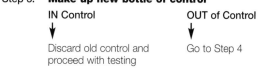

Step 2. **Inspect control for: Outdate (age), proper storage, correct lot number, signs of contamination.**

YES there is a problem   NO obvious explanation

↓   ↓

Make new control and retest   **RETEST**

                    ↓

          IN Control   OUT of Control

          ↓   ↓

          Proceed with   Go to Step 3
          testing

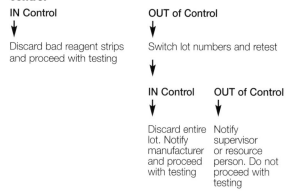

Step 3. **Make up new bottle of control**

IN Control   OUT of Control

↓   ↓

Discard old control and   Go to Step 4
proceed with testing

Step 4. **Open new can of reagent strips and test with new control**

IN Control   OUT of Control

↓   ↓

Discard bad reagent strips   Switch lot numbers and retest
and proceed with testing

                    ↓

          IN Control   OUT of Control

          ↓   ↓

          Discard entire   Notify
          lot. Notify   supervisor
          manufacturer   or resource
          and proceed   person. Do not
          with testing   proceed with
                      testing

Supervisors should consider urinalysis to be as vital as other areas of the clinical laboratory when appropriating continuing education dollars for reference books and attendance at local, regional, and national meetings.

Conclusion

Urinalysis is a multifaceted process that requires QC and QA measures both inside and outside the laboratory. Supervisors and laboratory directors must be concerned not only with minimum standards but also with the continual monitoring and incorporation of advances that can improve this commonly used test. Standardization of all in-laboratory aspects of the urinalysis procedure represents the only way in which subjectivity and variability can be eliminated, granting urinalysis improved status in laboratory testing.

References

BMC/Biodynamics: *Manufacturers Insert and Technical Bulletin.* Indianapolis, Indiana; BMC/Biodynamics, 1986. (BMC is now Roche.)

Clark DA: A laboratory quality control program that boosts technologists morale. *J Med Technol* 1985: 2:650:654.

College of American Pathologists: *Commission on Laboratory Accreditation. Inspection Checklist: Urinalysis Section III-A,* Skokie, IL; College of American Pathologists, Spring 1984.

Fuller CE, Threatte GA, Henry JB: Basic examination of urine. *Clinical Diagnosis and Management by Laboratory Methods,* 12th ed. Saunders, Philadelphia, 367-397, 2001.

ICL Scientific, Inc: *Technical Bulletin,* Fountain Valley, CA: ICL Scientific, 1982.

Ross DL, Neely AE: *Textbook of Urinalysis and Body Fluids.* Norwalk, Connecticut; Apple-Century Crofts, 1983.

Schumann GB, Schumann JL, Schweitzer SC: The urine sediment examination: A coordinated approach. *Lab Management* 21:45-48, 1983.

Schumann GB: Examination of urine, in Kaplan LA, Pesce AK (eds): *Clinical Chemistry: Theory, Analysis and Correlation.* St Louis; CV Mosby, 996-1031, 1984a.

Schumann GB, Schumann JL: *Manual of Cytodiagnostic Urinalysis.* Salt Lake City, Utah Cytodiagnostics, 1984b.

Schumann GB, Schumann JL, DeBelia C: Cytodiagnostic urinalysis: The method and its applications. *Lab Management* 1:36-40, 1985.

Schumann GB, Tebbs RD: Comparison of slides used for standardized routine microscopic urinalysis. *J Med Technol* 1986: 3: 54-58

Schweitzer SC, Schumann JL, Schumann GB: Quality assurance guidelines for the urinalyis laboratory. *J Med Technol* 3:567-571, 1986.

Stewart CE: The choice of a control material: Important factors. *J Med Technol* 1985: 2:637-654.

Strasinger SK: *Urinalysis and Body Fluids: A Self-Instructional Text,* Philadelphia: FA Davis, 1985.

Tetrault GA: Clinical laboratory quality assurance. *Clinical Diagnosis and Management by Laboratory Methods,* 12th ed. Saunders, Philadelphia, 148-156, 2001.

Travers EM, McClatchey KD: Basic laboratory management. *Clinical Laboratory Management,* 2nd ed. Lippincott Williams & Wilkins, Philadelphia, 3-11, 2002.

V-Tech Inc: *Count-10 Systems: Technical Bulletin,* Palm Desert, CA; V-Tech, 1983.

Whale Scientific: *Technical Bulletin.* Commerce City, CO. Whale Scientific, 1982.

Glossary

Acanthocyte: Erythrocyte characterized by irregularly speculated projections and associated with renal (glomerular) bleeding.

Acanthocyturia: Presence of acanthocytic erythrocyte in urine. A characteristic marker of glomerular bleeding.

Accuracy: Correctness of a test result; freedom from error or how close a test result is to the "true" or actual value.

Action Levels: (for hazardous substances) Exposures to specific hazardous chemicals that, while below the permissible exposure limit, still require that certain action take place under specific conditions (eg, medical surveillance or monitoring of the workplace).

Active Reabsorption: Reabsorption that requires an expenditure of energy for the analyte to be reabsorbed usually against a concentration gradient from a region of lower to one of high concentration.

Acute Glomerulonephritis (AGN), Postinfectious Glomerulonephritis: Glomerulonephritis of short duration that may occur 1 to 6 weeks after a streptococcal (usually Group A, β-hemolytic) infection.

Acute Tubular Necrosis (ATN): Disease clinically causing acute renal failure and cytologically characterized by the destruction of renal tubular epithelial cells and a reduced blood supply to the renal tubules.

Addis Count: Quantitative wet urine sediment test in which the number of erythrocytes, leukocytes, and casts are quantified in a timed urine specimen.

Aerosols: Infectious particles that are airborne; fine mist in which particles are dispersed.

Albumin: Simple protein that is water-soluble and coagulated by heat.

Albuminuria: Increased albumin in urine.

Aldosterone: Mineralocorticoid hormone released from the adrenal medulla that stimulates active absorption of sodium ion in exchange for potassium ion that is excreted by renal tubular cells (the sodium/potassium pump).

Amber: Term used to describe urine color; a dark yellow or orange-red color that may indicate a very concentrated urine specimen, or the presence of bilirubin or urobilin pigment.

Aminoaciduria: Excess of one or more amino acids in urine.

Amorphous Crystals: Shapeless, ill-defined crystals, usually phosphates or urates.

Amorphous Material: Crystalline material seen in the urine sediment as granules, without shape or form.

Antidiuretic Hormone (ADH): Pituitary hormone that decreases the production of urine by increasing the reabsorption of water by the renal tubules. Also called vasopressin.

Anisocytosis: Abnormal variability in cell size; often used in reference to erythrocyte morphology and abnormalities.

Anuria: Decrease in urine excretion to ≤100 mL/24 hr.

Artifact: Nonpathologic structures in urine sediment, often resulting from improper urine collection techniques, improper slide preparation, or extraneous sources of contamination.

Ascorbic Acid (Vitamin C): Strong reducing agent that acts as an interfering substance (resulting in delayed or false-negative results) in many reagent strip tests that utilize the release of oxygen and subsequent oxidation of chromogen.

Bacteriuria: Presence of unicellular microorganisms in urine.

Barrier Precautions: Personal protective devices (gloves, gowns) placed between blood or other potentially infectious body fluid specimen and the person handling the specimen to prevent transmission of the pathogenic agents borne by the specimen.

Bence-Jones Protein: Light chain immunoglobulin seen almost exclusively in urine of patients with multiple myeloma; coagulates at temperatures of 45 to 55°C and redissolves partially or completely on boiling.

Benedicts Test: Copper reduction test for reducing substances based on the reduction of cupric (copper II) ions to cuprous (copper I) ions in the presence of alkali and heat.

Bilirubin: Vivid yellow pigment; major by-product of normal red blood cell destruction. See also conjugated bilirubin, free (unconjugated) bilirubin.

Bilirubinuria: Presence of bilirubin in urine.

Biohazard Container: Special container to be used for disposal of all potentially infectious materials—blood, other body fluids, and tissues and disposable materials contaminated with them; containers should be tagged "biohazard" or bear the universal symbol.

Birefringence: Ability of some crystals or objects to rotate or polarize light so they are visible when viewed with crossed polarizing filters.

Bladder: Elastic muscular sac which collects and stores urine until it can be voided.

Bowman's Capsule: See glomerular capsule.

Brightfield Microscope: Illumination system used in the common clinical microscope.

Calculus: Concretion in the urinary system or other tissues, usually composed of mineral salts. Its formation is referred to as lithiasis.

Carcinoma In Situ: Morphologically recognizable pervasive stage of certain malignant epithelial neoplasms (carcinoma).

Carnoy's Fixative: Fixative with acetic acid used primarily for lysing red blood cells.

Casts: Cylindrical structure resulting from protein precipitation where there is decreased urine flow. Casts are formed in the lumen of the nephron's distal convoluted tubule or in the collecting ducts.

Catheterization: Passage of a thin, flexible tube into the bladder or ureter for the drainage of urine.

Catheterized Urine Specimen: Urine specimen obtained by the introduction of a catheter into the urinary bladder by way of the urethra.

Cell Block: Method used to concentrate cells or small tissue fragments for histologic examination.

Centrifugation: Concentration of elements in fluid by centrifugal force.

Chemical Hygiene Plan: Mandated as part of the OSHA hazard communication standard. This plan must be in place in the laboratory to inform workers and carry out implementation of safety practices necessary to protect the workers from potential health hazards associated with laboratory chemicals in use.

Clean-Catch (Midstream) Urine Specimen: Urine specimen collected during the middle of a flow of urine, after the urinary opening has been carefully cleansed. The type of urine collection used for bacterial culture.

Clinical Laboratory Improvement Act of 1976 (CLIA '76): Act providing for the licensing of laboratories that accept specimens for testing from across state lines (interstate commerce), generally large hospital and reference laboratories.

Clinical Laboratory Improvement Amendments of 1988 (CLIA '88): Standards set for all laboratories to ensure quality patient care; provisions include requirements for quality control and assurance, for the use of proficiency tests, and for certain levels of personnel to perform and supervise work done in all clinical laboratories. Applies to any entity that performs testing on material derived from humans for the purpose of diagnosis, assessment, or treatment.

Clue Cell: Squamous epithelial cells covered (encrusted) with *Garderella vaginalis*; indicates bacterial vaginosis.

Collecting Tubules: Relatively large, straight renal tubules after the distal convoluted tubules of the nephron which connect individual nephrons at various intervals and funnel urine into the renal pelvis, the site of final concentration of urine under the control of ADH (vasopressin).

Compensated Polarized Light: Modification of the normal brightfield microscope in which two crossed polarizing filters plus a first-order red compensator or filter are inserted to observe the presence or absence and type of birefringence. Especially useful in identification of synovial fluid crystals in the clinical laboratory.

Confirmatory Test: Method used to demonstrate the accuracy or correctness of a procedure, with at least the same or better specificity, based on a different principle, with equal or better sensitivity than the original test.

Conjugated Bilirubin, Bilirubin Glucuronide, Direct Bilirubin: Bilirubin that has been made water soluble by chemically bonding with glucuronide by the Kupffer cells of the liver. Once conjugated, increased levels of bilirubin in the blood can be filtered through the kidney and found in the urine.

Continuous Quality Improvement (CQI): Ongoing process to ensure that quality outcomes are attained to satisfy the needs of the patient, involves the philosophy of TQM. See also Total Quality Management.

Control Specimen (Solution): Material or solution with a known concentration of the analyte(s) being measured; used for quality control in which the test result for the control specimen must be within certain limits in order for the unknown values run in the same "batch" or time frame to be considered reportable.

Cortex (Renal): Outer layer of the kidney made up of the glomerular portions of the nephron and the proximal convoluted tubules.

Crenated (RBCs): Red blood cells or erythrocytes showing spicules or projections on the surface this notched, shriveled surface results from loss of fluid from the red cell into the urine caused by hypertonicity. Considered a specific type of dysmorphic erythrocyte.

Critical (Panic) Value: Dangerously abnormal test results (high or low) that are used to guide emergency notification of clinical teams. Accrediting agencies require that clinical laboratories establish a list of critical limits to suit their needs and to devolop formal notification policies with documentation of such communication. These values reflect medical decision levels for emergency patient evaluation and optimization points for critical care.

Coverslipping: Method of preserving a cytologic or histologic slide preparation using a solvent-based adhesive mounting and a coverglass.

Creatinine: Nitrogenous end product of creatine metabolism; normally found in blood and urine in small amounts (0.02 g/kg).

Crystals, Abnormal: Urinary crystals of metabolic or iatrogenic origin that are generally of pathologic significance and require further if possible chemical confirmation.

Crystals, Urinary: Urinary crystals that may be found in benign urine specimens of an acid or alkaline pH; generally they are physiologic rather than pathologic and can be reported on the basis of morphologic appearance and amount.

Cylindroid: Hyaline cast with one end that tapers off into a tail or point; clinically equivalent to and reported as a hyaline cast.

Crystalluria: Presence of crystals in urine.

Cylindruria: Presence of casts in urine.

Cystitis: Inflammation of the bladder characterized by symptoms of urgency, frequency, dysuria, and/or nocturia.

Cytocentrifugation: Method of concentrating cellular material on a small, confined area of a slide.

Cytodiagnostic Urinalysis: Specialized cytologic urine test combining both physicochemical assessments with concentrated Papanicolaou-stained urine sediment examination.

Cytomegalic Inclusion Disease: Viral condition (cytomegalovirus—CMV) affecting the kidney and other organs, causing cells to enlarge with intranuclear inclusions.

Diabetes Mellitus: Chronic metabolic syndrome of impaired carbohydrate, fat, and protein metabolism that is secondary to insufficiency of insulin secretion or to the inhibition of the activity of insulin, characterized by increased concentration of glucose in the blood and urine.

Diazo Reaction: Coupling of a diazonium salt with another aromatic ring to give an azo dye.

Dipstick Urinalysis: Chemical urine test for the detection of albumin, glucose, ketone, bilirubin, hemoglobin, bacteria, leukocytes, and other chemical constituents.

Distal Convoluted Tubule: Convoluted tubules of the nephron furthest from the glomerulus where final reabsorption of sodium (maintaining water and electrolyte balance) and removal of excess acid (maintaining acid base balance) occurs.

Diuretic: Agent that promotes the secretion of urine.

Documentation: A written record. In the labortoary this includes all personnel records, policies and procedures, quality assurance measures, incidents, and corrective actions.

Dysmorphic (RBCs): Having structural defects or fragmentation.

Dysmorphic Erythrocyturia: Presence of fragmented erythrocytes in urine sediment indicating renal (glomerular or tubular) hematuria.

Dysuria: Painful urination.

Edema: Swelling due to excessive fluid retention. Associated with renal (glomular) bleeding.

Ehrlich's Aldehyde Reaction: Reaction of urobilinogen, porphobilinogen, and other Ehrlich-reactive compounds with p-dimethylaminobenzaldehyde in concentrated hydrochloric acid to form a colored aldehyde.

Eosinophil: Granulated white blood cell with a nucleus that has one or two lobes connected by a thread of chromatin. The cytoplasm contains coarse eosinophilic granules.

Epithelial Cell: Cells which compose the epidermis of the skin and line the surface layer of mucous and serous membranes.

Erythrocyte: Red blood cell.

Erythrocyturia: Presence of RBCs in urine.

Erythrophagocytosis: Ingestion of red blood cells by macrophages.

Exfoliate: To peel or slough off, such as the process by which epithelial cells lining the urinary system are continually sloughed off and replaced.

Exogenous: Coming from or being introduced into a specimen from the outside, such as contaminants from powder in gloves.

Extravascular Fluid: Liquid within the body found outside of any blood or lymphatic vessel.

First Morning Urine Specimen: First urine voided in the morning. It is generally the most concentrated specimen of the day because less fluid or water is excreted during the night, yet the kidney has maintained excreted during the night, yet the kidney has maintained excretion of a constant concentration of solid or dissolved substances.

Fistula: Abnormal connection such as a fistula between the colon and urinary tract.

Free Bilirubin, Unconjugated Bilirubin: Water-insoluble form of bilirubin that must be carried through the blood stream as a bilirubin-albumin complex. Because of its insolubility, this form of bilirubin cannot be excreted by the kidney and is not found in the urine.

Fixation: Process by which living tissues or cells are rapidly killed to preserve structures present in life.

Funguria: Presence of fungus in urine.

Galactosemia: Inherited, autosomal-recessive disorder of galactose metabolism, characterized by a deficiency of the enzyme galactose-1-phosphated uridyl transferase, resulting in increased levels of galactose in the blood (galactosemia) and urine (glactosuria).

Ghost or Shadow Cell: Red cells that have burst, releasing hemoglobin, leaving only the red cell membrane; visualization enhanced by phase-contrast microscopy.

Glitter Cells: Pale staining, swollen, and degenerated neutrophils found in dilute urine, with cytoplasmic granules that exhibit a characteristic brownian movement.

Glomerular Filtrate: Constituent of blood which pass through the glomerular basement membrane and enter the renal tubule.

Glomeruli: Coils of blood vessels projecting into the expanded end of the capsule of each of the uriniferous tubules of the kidney.

Glomerulonephritis: Inflammation of glomeruli causing increased permeability to blood and protein.

Glomerulus: Tuft or cluster of blood vessels, found in the renal nephron. Urine formation begins at the glomerulus.

Glucose Oxidase: Enzyme that oxidizes glucose to gluconic acid while reducing atmospheric oxygen to hydrogen peroxide.

Glycosuria: Presence of abnormal amounts of glucose in urine.

Gram-Staining Reaction: Using the gram-staining method, microorganisms retaining the violet (purple) color of the primary stain (crystal violet-iodine complex) are considered *Gram-positive*; microorganisms having the red-pink color of the counterstain(safranin) are considered *Gram-negative*.

Hansel's Stain: Stain containing methylene blue and eosin-Y in methanol; used to stain for the presence of eosinophils.

Haptoglobin: Plasma protein that binds and carries free hemoglobin in the bloodstream. When haptoglobin is saturated, free hemoglobin is filtered into the urine.

Hazard Identification System: Symbol that provides, at a glance, information about potential health, flammability, and chemical reactivity for potential hazards from materials used in the laboratory; a larger diamond-shaped figure made up of four smaller diamonds, one red, one blue, one yellow and one white, each indicating the particular hazardous information pertaining to the chemical in question.

Hematuria: Abnormal presence of blood in urine.

Hemoglobin: Oxygen-carrying, iron-containing pigment of red blood cells.

Hemoglobinuria: Presence of free hemoglobin in urine.

Hemolytic Jaundice, Prehepatic Jaundice: Jaundice that results from increased destruction of red cells in blood (intravascular hemolysis).

Hemosiderin: Iron-rich pigment that is a product of red cell hemolysis: storage from of iron in the bone marrow. In urine, hemosiderin is seen as iron-containing granules that may occur after a hemolytic episode. Stain blue with Prussian blue stain for iron (Rous test).

Hemosiderinuria: Presence of hemosiderin in the urine.

Hepatic Jaundice, Hepatocellular jaundice: Jaundice resulting from conditions that affect the liver cells directly, such as viral or toxic hepatitis.

High-Power Examination: Usually a 40× magnification objective and 10× occular giving a total magnification of 400×; used for more detailed examination of wet preparations.

Histiocyte: Tissue cell that is a part of the reticuloendothelial system.

Hoesch Test: Inverse Ehrlich's aldehyde reaction used to detect porphobilinogen in urine.

Hyaline Cast: Transparent cast composed of mucoprotein.

Hydrometer: Instrument used for determining the specific gravity of a fluid.

Hyperchromasia: Excessive pigmentation; generally applies to a cell nucleus which stains darkly because it is filled with particles of chromatin.

Hypertonic: Solution with a greater osmotic pressure than a comparable solution.

Illeal Conduit: Surgically constructed sac made from a loop of small intestine, which functions as a bladder, usually after cytectomy for bladder cancer.

Insulin: Hormone that has the effect of lowering the blood glucose concentration by promoting transport and entry of glucose into muscle cells and other tissues.

Interstitial Nephritis: Inflammation of the interstitial tissue of the kidney, including the tubules. May be acute or chronic. Acute interstitial nephritis is an immunologic, adverse reaction to certain drugs, often sulfonamide or methicillin.

Iris Diaphragm: Part of the microscope located at the bottom of the Abbe condenser, under the lens but within the condenser body, controls the amount of light passing through the material under observation, can opened or closed to adjust contrast.

Jaundice: Increase in the concentration of free or conjugated bilirubin in the blood (serum) with accumulation of bilirubin in the body tissues. See also Hemolytic jaundice, hepatic jaundice, and obstructive jaundice.

Ketogenic Diet: Diet that consists of more than 1.5 g or fat per 1.0 g of carbohydrate; results in ketosis.

Ketosis: Increased concentration of ketones in the blood (ketonemia) and urine (ketonuria).

Ketone: Any compound containing the carbonyl group C=O and having hydrocarbon groups attached to the carbonyl carbon.

Ketonuria: Presence of ketone in urine.

Kidneys: Pair of bean-shaped organs which maintain homeostasis by filtering blood, forming urine that contains the end products of metabolism.

Leukocyte Esterase: Enzyme present in the azurophilic or primary granules of the granulocytic leukocytes. Presence of this enzyme in urine (leukocyte esterasuria) indicates urinary tract infection of inflammation.

Lithiasis: Kidney stone (calculus) formation.

Lipid: Fat or fat-like substance which is insoluable in water and is utilized as a fuel source.

Loop of Henle: The U-shaped portion of the nephron between the proximal and distal convoluted tubules, consisting of a thin descending (concentrating) limb and a thick ascending (diluting) limb.

Low-Power Examination: Usually a 10× magnification objective and and 10× ocular, giving a total magnification of 100 times; used for the initial scanning and observation in most clinical microscopic work.

Lower Urinary Tract: Portion of the urinary tract excluding the kidney (eg, the ureters, bladder, and urethra). Lower urinary tract infections are generally infections of the bladder, also known as cystitis.

Lymphocyte: Mononuclear white blood cell produced in lymphoid tissue.

Macroscopic Urinalysis: Physical and chemical analyses of urine.

Maltese Cross: White cross on a black background, characteristic of cholesterol ester droplets in urine or other body fluids, viewed with polarized light. Must not be confused with granules of starch.

Material Safety Data Sheets (MSDS): In formation about the hazards of each chemical are provided by the supplier or manufacturer of the chemical; any hazardous chemicals used in the laboratory should be accompanied by this information.

Medulla: (Renal) Part of the parenchyma of the kidney, beneath the cortices, including the renal pyramids and columns; includes the loop of Henle and collecting tubules.

Melanin: Dark amorphous pigment of the skin, hair, and various tumors. It is produced by polymerization of oxidation products of tyorsine and dihydroxyphenol compounds and contains carbon, hydrogen, nitrogen, oxygen, and often sulfur.

Microalbuminuria: Consistent passage of very small amounts of protein as albumin into the urine. Associated with the early development of nephropathy in patients with diabetes mellitus.

Microscopic Urinalysis: Microscopic analysis of urine sediment to identify cells, organisms, casts, crystals and other formed elements.

Midstream Urine Specimen: Urine specimen collected during the middle of a flow of urine; used for routine urinalysis.

Monocyte: Large, mononuclear white blood cell found in the peripheral blood and urine.

Myoglobin: Coagulable globulin which stores oxygen found in muscle tissue.

Myoglobinuria: Presence of myoglobin in the urine.

Neoplasia: The formation of a new, abnormal lesion which grows at the expense of other tissues.

Nephritis: Inflammation of the kidney which may involve the glomeruli, tubules, or interstitium, either singly or simultaneously.

Nephron: Structural and functional unit of the kidney in which urine is formed.

Nephrotic syndrome: Glomerular disorder characterized by proteinuria, lipiduria, hypoproteinemia, and edema.

Neutrophil: White blood cell containing three to five lobed nuclei with neutrophilic granules in the cytoplasm.

Nidus: Point of origin, focus or nucleus; such as the nidus for urinary stone formation.

Nitrite: Salt of nitrous acid formed by the bacterial reduction of nitrate to nitrite.

Nuclear:Cytoplasmic Ratio: The relationship between the nuclear area of the cell and the area of the cytoplasm.

Obstructive Jaundice, Posthepatic Jaundice: Jaundice resulting from blockage of the normal outflow of conjugated bilirubin from the liver into the intestine.

Occult blood: Hidden blood, not observable by the naked eye, but requireing use of a chemical test to be detected.

Occupational Safety and Health Act (OSHA): Legislation of 1970 that set a system of safeguards for the health and safety of workers in the United States.

Oil Red O Stain: Stain which detects the presence of lipid by staining it bright red.

Oliguria: Diminished urine formation relative to fluid intake.

Organized Sediment: Biologic portion of the urine sediment including cells derived from blood, epithelial cells, other cell forms, and fat of biologic origin.

OSHA Standard: Hazard Communication; designed to ensure that all laboratory workers are fully aware of possible hazardous situations present in their workplace includes the implementation of a Chemical Hygiene Plan. This is also known as the Right to Know rule.

Osmolality: Measurement of the number of solute particles per unit solvent.

Oval Fat Bodies: Renal epithelial cells (also macrophages or histocytes) filled with fat droplets (cholesterol or neutral fat); associated with the presence of free fat globules and fatty casts.

Papanicolaou Stain: Polychromatic stain useful in the assessment of benign, malignant, cellular, and noncellular consitituents of many body sites.

Parasite: Organism that lives upon or within another organism, deriving its nourishment for survival without compensation to the host.

Parlodion Fixative: Plastic adhesive dissolved in absoute ethanol; used on glass slides to prevent cell loss.

Passive Reabsorption: Reabsorption that does not require the expenditure of energy; the analyte moves passively down a concentration gradient, from a region of higher to a region of lower concentration.

Pathologic Cast: Formed tubular urinary structure consisting of precipitated proteins, indicating stasis and disease involving the kidney.

Perineal Contamination: Contamination originating from the perineum; generally from the foreskin, vagina, or anus.

Permissive Exposure Limits (PEL): As designated by OSHA laboratory workers must not be exposed to hazardous chemical substances in excess of certain levels—the PEL; this information must be part of the Chemical Hygiene Plan for the laboratory, and the workers must be informed about the permissible exposure levels of the various hazardous chemicals being used.

Peroxidase: Enzyme that catalyzes release of free oxygen from hydrogen peroxide. Peroxidase activity for the heme portion of the hemoglobin molecule is the basis of the reagent-strip test for blood.

Periodic Acid-Schiff (PAS): Stain used for the identification of fungi, mucin, glycogen, and carbohydrates.

Personal Protective Equipment (PPE): Specialized clothing or protective varriers worn or used for protection against a hazardous substance or agent.

pH: Expression of the hydrogen ion concentration (acidity or alkalinity) of a solution

Phase-Contrast Microscope: Microscope illumination system that used a special condenser with an annular diaphragm with a matched absorption ring in the corresponding objective. Used to give additional contrast in wet preparations; especially useful for observing the urine sediment.

Phenazopyridine (Pyridium): Azo-containing compound often used as a urine analgesic to reduce pain in cystitis or other urinary tract infections. Azo-containing compounds are a common cause of interference (masking or false-positive reactions) in urine reagent strip tests.

Phenyketonuria: Phenylpyruvic acid in urine; an inborn error of metabolism.

Phosphate: Any ester or salt of phosphoric acid.

Physical Properties: In urinalysis, includes color, transparency (or clarity), odor, form, volume, and specific gravity of a urine specimen.

Physiologic Cast: Precipitated urinary proteins which gel in the tubules; commonly found following strenuous exercise and dehydration.

Poikilocytosis: Abnormal variability in the shape of erythrocytes.

Point of Care (POC) Testing : Tests that can be performed at the patient's bedside or patient care unit, thus giving a result more quickly by eliminating time for specimen handling and transportation to a distant centralized laboratory site. Generally, the tests that can be completed within a 5 minute total turnaround time (TAT) are candidates for POC testing (see Total Turnaround Time).

Polarized Light: Light that is propagated in such a way that the radiation waves occur in only one direction in the vibration plane and not at random. In the microscope, light is polarized by adding a polarizing filter.

Polarizing Mircrscope: Microscope illumination system that employs two polarizing lenses, which are crossed, extinguishing passage of light through the microscope; used to detect objects or crystals that bend or polarize light, making them visible when viewed with crossed polarizing filters.

Polyuria: Excessive elimination of large amounts of urine relative to fluid intake.

Porphobilinogen: Colorless precursor of porphyrins, a group of compounds utilized in the synthesis of hemoglobin.

Postinfectious Glomerulonephritis: See acute glomerulonephritis and glomerulonephritis.

Porphyrins: Group of iron-free or magnesium-free pyrrole derivatives that occur universally in cells. They constitute the basis of the respiratory pigments in animals and plants.

Precision: Repeatability or reproducibility of a test result; a measure of the closeness of repeated test results on the same sample.

Proficiency Testing (PT): Program under which samples are sent to a group of laboratories for analysis; results are compared with those of other laboratories participating in the program. Included as a component of quality assurance programs to establish quality control between laboratories.

Prostate: Glandular organ that surrounds the neck of the gladder and the proximal portion of the male urethra; its main function is the production of prostatic fluid, a component of semen.

Protein: Complex nitrogenous compound in plants and animals comprised of amino acid combinations which are essential for tissue growth and repair.

Protein Error of pH Indicators: Phenomenon in which at a fixed pH, certain pH indicators will show one color in the presence of protein and another color in its absence.

Proteinuria: Excessive amounts of protains, usually albumin, in the urine.

Proximal Convoluted Tubule: Convoluted tubules of the nephron closest to the glomerular capsule in which about 80% of the fluid and electryolytes filtered through the glomerulus are reabsorbed.

Pseudocast: Cast-like structures which simulate the appearance of true casts but do not contain hyaline or granular matrix.

Pseudohyphae: Elongated cell forms of yeast, such as *Candida* sp., that resemble mycelia (hyphae), the thread-like filaments that make up most fungi.

Pyelonephritis: Inflammation of the kidney and renal pelvis; also known as tubulointerstitial inflammation (TII). Acute pyelonephritis is usually the result of an infection that ascends from the lower urinary tract to the kidney. Chronic pyelonephritis develops slowly after bacterial infection of the kidney (usually associated with obstruction) and may progress to renal failure.

Pyuria: Presence of an abnormal number of WBCs (pus) in urine.

Quality Assurance (QA): Comprehensive set of policies, procedures, and practices in place and used to make certain that the laboratory's reported results are reliable and can be used by the physician to diagnose and or treat the patient. QA includes all aspects of the laboratory (technical and nontechnical) to prevent errors and ensure accuracy of test results. It includes preanalytical, analytical, and postanalytical factors such as record keeping, calibration and maintenance of equipment, quality control, proficiency testing, and training.

Quality Control (QC): Part of quality assurance utilizing a set of laboratory procedures designed to ensure that a test method is working properly and meets the diagnostic needs of the physician. QC makes use of control solutions or specimens and includes testing of control samples, charting the results, and analyzing them statistically.

Random Voided Urine Specimen: Voided urine specimen obtained at any point of a 24-hour period.

Reagent-strip (Dipstick) Testing: Use of a chemical test strip to determine whether pathologic concentrations of various substances are present in the urine.

Refractive Index: Ratio of the velocity of light in air to the velocity of light in solution; used to measure concentrating ability in urine.

Refractometer: Instrument which measures the refractive index of a solution.

Reliability: Ability of a laboratory assay to produce consistent results when testing is repeated successfully. Includes accuracy and precision.

Renal Epithelial Cells, Renal Tubular Epithelium (RTE): Epithelial cells originating from (lining) the tubules of the kidney from the proximal to the collecting tubules; Appearance varies and depends on actual site of origin.

Renal Epithelial Fragment: Fragment of renal epithelial cells originating from the collecting duct, three or more attached renal cells of collecting duct origin.

Renal Failure Cast: Synonym for broad waxy cast; clinically represents serious pathology and chronic renal failure.

Renal Plasma Threshold: Concentration of an analyte that can be completely reabsorbed from the glomerular filtrate. When the plasma concentraton of an analyte exceeds this value, it will remain in the glomerular filtrate and be excreted in the urine.

Renal Tubular Fat: See oval fat bodies.

Renal Tubular Injury: Abnormal or increased exfolioation of renal tubular epithelial cells of convoluted, collecting duct, or necrotic origin.

Rhabdomyolysis: Acute destruction of muscle fibers.

Right to Know Rule: OSHA standard whereby all persons working in the area must be made fully aware of possible hazardous situations present in their workplace that might be detrimental to their safety and well-being.

Rous Test: Wet staining procedure for hemosiderin granules in urine sediment utilizing a Prussian blue reaction for iron.

Safety Manual: Manual readily available to all persons working in the laboratory that includes current information about all safety practices and precautions, anything that could pose a potential safety hazard for persons in the laboratory must be described in this manual and each worker in the laboratory must be familiar with its contents.

Sensitivity: Minimum detectable level of an analyte in a given laboratory procedure or test. Statistically, the proportion of subjects with a positive diagnostic test result in a diseased population, expressed as a percentage.

Sequential Collection: Samples are collected in order (sequence) with the order of collection noted on the specimen container.

Specific Gravity: Weight of a given volume of solution compared to an equal volume of water at a specified temperature.

Specificity: Refers to what is actually being measured in a given labortatory test. Statistically, the proportion of subjects with a negative diagnostic test in a population without the disease, expressed as a percentage.

Squamous Epithelial Cells: Large, flat, scalelike epithelial cells that line the female urethra and trigone, distal portion of the male urethra, and female vagina.

Staghorm Calculi: Urinalry calculi (stones) that fill the renal collecting system; especially characteristic of cystine, struvite (triple phosphate), and uric acid.

Starch: In urine sediment, refers to cornstarch (a carbohydrate that is commonly used to line surgical or barrier protective gloves); a common urinary contaminant different from talc. Polarizes as a maltese cross.

Sternheimer-Malbin Stain: Crystal violet and safranin supravital stain used in wet urinalysis; provides additional contrast for some cells and casts.

Talc, Talcum: Hydrated magnesium silicate; a chunky, irregular crystal formerly used to line surgical gloves; a possible urinary contaminant. Talc is not starch.

Tamm-Horsfall Protein: Glycoprotein (mucoprotein) secreted by renal tubular cells and not derived from blood or plama; forms the matrix of urinary casts.

Target Cell: Abnormal erythrocyte with a darker-staining outer rim surrounded by a lighter-staining rim, resembling a target or bull's eye.

Telescopic Sediment: Urine sediment seen after a period of renal shutdown, where a range of casts from hyaline to waxy with intermediate stages are seen.

Toluidine Blue: Supravital stain that is easily prepared in the laboratory; useful in the brightfield examination of urine sediment and to assess nuclear features of cells.

Total (or Therapeutic) Turnaround Time (TTAT): Time starting with that point where the physician determines a need for a particular laboratory value for a diagnosis or treatment plan to when the physician has the value in hand on which to act.

Tonicity: Effective osmotic pressure equivalent.

Total Quality Management (TQM): Design of systems and procedures used to ensure that quality is attained throughout an institution; emphasizes teamwork or performance, rather than individual or departmental performance. Patient satisfaction is the goal for a health care institution for the clinical laboratory; an example of TQM is the improvement or reporting results of tests so they have a greater impact on patient care.

Transitional Epithelial Cells: Urothelial cells; stratified epithelial lining of the urinary tract from the pelvis of the kidney to the bases of the bladder (trigone) in females and the proximal part of the urethra in males. In the urinary tract, urothelial cells originate in structures located between structures lined by squamous and renal epithelial cells.

Transparency: In urinalysis, an assessment of the degree of clarity, or cloudiness, of a urine specimen: a description of the amount of solid material suspended in the urine.

Trichomonas: Motile protozoan parasite that may infect the vagina, urethra, periurethral glands, bladder, and prostate. May be seen in the urine sediment, but usually searched for in wet preparations of direct swabs from the vagina or urethra.

Trigone: Triangular structure; the base of the urinary bladder.

Tubular Reabsorption: Selective reabsorption of substances in the glomerular filtrate into the boodstream across the renal tubular epithelial cells.

Tubular Secretion: Secretion by the renal tubular epithelium of substances including metabolic wastes from the vasa recta into the lumen of the renal tubules through the renal tubular epithelial cells

Turnaround Time (TAT): For the physician, the time between which a laboratory test is first desired, ordered, or collected, and results are obtained. For the laboratory, generally the time between receipt of the specimen in the laboratory, and the reporting of results.

Ultrafiltrate of Plasma: Filtrate of plasma across a membrane, where extremely small particles such as proteins are restricted or filtered—essentially the filtrate contains the same composition as the plasma.

Unconjugated Bilirubin: See free bilirubin.

Universal Precautions: Includes a system of recommended safety practices and policies (infection control) used for handling all biologic (patient) specimens. Potential infectivity of any patient body fluid (including blood) is unknown, and therefore all blood and body fluid specimens are considered to be equally infectious (also known as universal blood and body fluid precautions).

Unorganized Sediment: Chemical portion of the urine sediment, consisting of crystals and amorphous deposits of chemicals.

Upper Urinary Tract: Generally the kidney and renal pelvis.

Urea: Primary end product of protein metabolism. The result of amino acid and protein breakdown.

Ureters: Two narrow, muscular tubes that actively transport urine from the kidneys to the bladder.

Urethra: Membranous canal which conducts urine to the outside of the body.

Urinalysis (Wet, Routine, Basic): Testing of urine with procedures commonly performed in an expeditious, reliable, and cost-effective manner in clinical laboratories. Includes the physical, chemical, and microscopic analysis of urine.

Urinary System: Consists of two kidneys and two ureters plus the bladder and urethra.

Urine Sediment: Any solid material that is suspended in the voided urine specimen. Includes cells, casts, crystals, amorphous deposits of chemicals, and other formed elements.

Urinometer: Specialized hydrometer calibrated to ensure specific gravity of urine at a given temperature. Measurement of specific gravity by urinometer is considered inaccurate and discouraged by NCCLS.

Urobilinogen: Colorless compound derived from the reduction of conjugated bilirubin by intestinal bacteria.

Urochrome: Primary pigment of urine derived from urobilin.

Uroerythrin: Red pigment; present in small amounts in normal urine.

Variance, Error: General term describing the factors of fluctuations that affect the measurement of a substance.

Viral Hepatitis: Inflammation of the liver caused by hepatitis virus.

Virus: Self-replicating parasitic organism consisting of a core nucleic acid enveloped by a protein coating.

Waived Tests: Set of eight specific tests and methodologies under CLIA '88 that are exempt from proficiency testing regulations. Laboratories performing only waived tests must obtain a Certificate of Waiver from the Department of Health and Human Services.

Wet Urinalysis: Screening or frontline urine test combining both physicochemical assessments and a wet unstained urine sediment examination.

Yeast: Unicellular fungal, nucleated microorganism that reproduces by budding; capable of fermenting carbohydrates.

Urinary System Disorders: Algorithms and Correlations

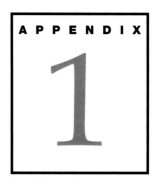

APPENDIX

1

Figure 1. Common Clinical Signs and Associated Conditions for Wet Urinalysis Testing

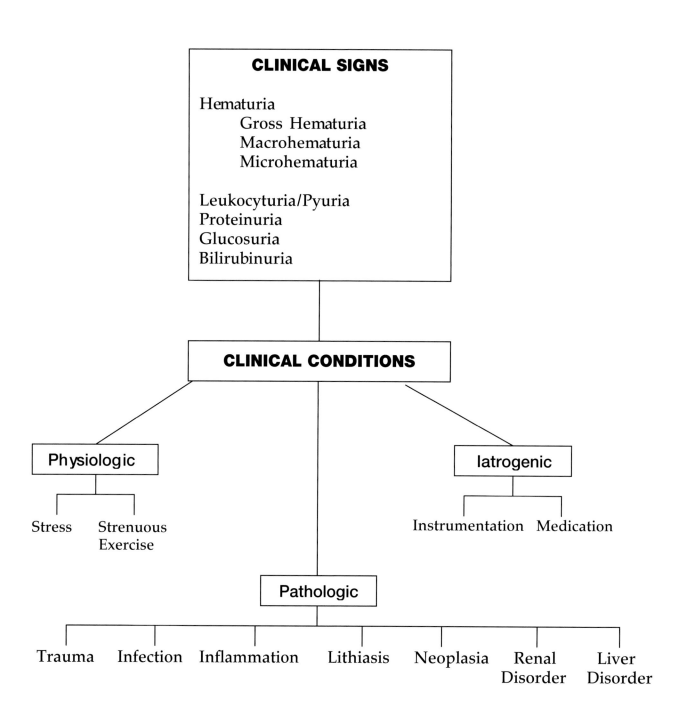

Figure 2. Algorithm and Correlations for Dipstick (Macroscopic) Hematuria

---

CLINICAL CONDITIONS:

Physiologic		Pathologic			
(Stress, Exercise)	Infection	Inflammation	Lithiasis	Neoplasia	Renal

Case Correlative

Examples:	Case #1			Case #2	Case #3	Case #5
					Case #4	

URINALYSIS FINDINGS:

Physical
  Color   ← ——— Yellow ——————————————— Amber ———→

Chemistry
  Dipstick   ← ——————————— 1–4+ Blood ——————————→
  Proteins   ← ——————— Variable ————————————————→

Cells
  RBCs   ←— Dys RBCs → ←———— Iso RBCs ———→   Dys RBCs
  WBCs   ←————— 1–4+ WBCs —————————→
  RTCs   Present

Casts   ←— Physiologic →   ← Pathologic →

Crystals   Occ

Concretions   Present

Microbiology   > 2+ Bacteria
                      > 2+ Fungi
                      Parasites

Epithelial Abnormalities   Abnormal   Suspect
                                                  cell   renal
                                                  and/or   fragment
                                                  fragment

---

dys=dysmorphic   iso=isomorphic   occ=occasional   RTC=renal tubular cell

CASE #1

HEMATURIA—PHYSIOLOGIC

AGE N/A
SEX N/A

SPECIMEN TYPE Random void

CLINICAL INFORMATION: Asymptomatic microhematuria.

MACROSCOPIC DESCRIPTION:
Color: Yellow *Clarity:* Clear *Specific Gravity:* 1.015 *Volume:* 80 mL

URINE CHEMISTRY:
Reagent Strip:
   pH 5   Blood (1+) Protein NEG Glucose NEG Ketones NEG
   Leukocytes NEG Nitrite NEG Bilirubin NEG Urobilinogen NEG

Confirmatory Studies: SSA <5 mg/dL Ictotest _____ Clinitest _____

MICROSCOPIC EVALUATION:
Background: Clean
   Crystals :
   Other (specify):

Erythrocytes: (8)/HPF
   Isomorphic /(Dysmorphic)

Leukocytes: ____ /HPF

Micro-organisms: Bacteria
   Fungus
   Parasites

Epithelial cells: Squamous
   Urothelial
   Renal

Casts: _____/LPF:

   Physiologic:
   —— Hyaline
   —— Granular

   Pathologic:
   —— Broad
   —— Fatty
   —— Cellular (RBC, WBC, RTC)
   —— Blood (heme-granular)
   —— Waxy

Lipid: Noncellular
   Cellular

Epithelial fragments:
Epithelial abnormalities:

INTERPRETATION:

Mild renal bleeding.

Comment: Mild renal bleeding is often related to stress and exercise.

RECOMMENDATIONS:
___ Microbiologic studies
___ Cytodiagnostic urinalysis
___ Renal function test

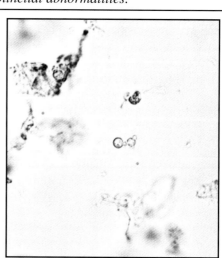

Wet Urinalysis

84

AGE __45__
SEX __F__   SPECIMEN TYPE __Random void__

CLINICAL INFORMATION: Back pain, microhematuria.

MACROSCOPIC DESCRIPTION:
Color: __Yellow__   *Appearance:* __Clear__   *Specific Gravity:* __1.010__   *Volume:* __40__ mL

URINE CHEMISTRY:
Reagent Strip:
    pH __5__   Blood __Trace__   Protein __NEG__   Glucose __NEG__   Ketones __NEG__
    Leukocytes __NEG__ Nitrite __NEG__   Bilirubin __NEG__   Urobilinogen __NEG__

Confirmatory Studies: SSA __< 5 mg/dL__

MICROSCOPIC EVALUATION:
Background: Moderately Dirty   *Casts:* _____ /LPF:
    Crystals (Calcium Oxalate, Calcium Monohydrate)
    Other (specify): (Concretions)   Physiologic:
                        ——— Hyaline
Erythrocytes: __3__ /HPF   ——— Granular
    (Isomorphic)/ Dysmorphic
                        Pathologic:
Leukocytes: __0__ /HPF   ——— Broad
                        ——— Fatty
Micro-organisms: Bacteria   ——— Cellular (RBC, WBC, RTC)
              Fungus   ——— Blood (heme-granular)
              Parasites   ——— Waxy

Epithelial cells: Squamous   *Lipid:*   Noncellular
              Urothelial   Cellular
              Renal
                        Epithelial fragments:

                        Epithelial abnormalities:

INTERPRETATION:
Crystalluria and concretions present. Suspect
microurolithiasis.

Comment: ————————————————

RECOMMENDATIONS:
    _____ Microbiologic studies
    __X__ Cytodiagnostic urinalysis
    _____ Renal function test
    __X__ Other: __Stone Risk Assessment__

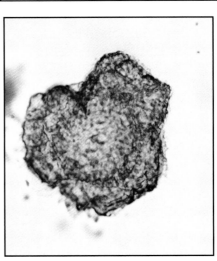

Appendix 1: Algorithms and Correlations

AGE __60__
SEX __M__   **SPECIMEN TYPE** __Catheterized__

CLINICAL INFORMATION: Hematuria, chronic cystitis and BPH.

MACROSCOPIC DESCRIPTION:
Color: __Yellow__   *Clarity :* __Slightly Cloudy__   *Specific Gravity:* __1.015__   *Volume:* __20__ ml

URINE CHEMISTRY:
Reagent Strip:
    pH __7.5__   Blood (2+)   Protein (1+ (30 mg/dL))   Glucose __NEG__   Ketones __NEG__
    Leukocytes (Trace)   Nitrite __NEG__   Bilirubin __NEG__   Urobilinogen __NEG__

Confirmatory Studies: SSA (40 mg/dL)   Ictotest _____   Clinitest _____   _____

MICROSCOPIC EVALUATION:
Background: **Slightly Dirty**   *Casts:* _____ /LPF:
   Crystals:
   Other (specify):   Physiologic:
                        ——— Hyaline
Erythrocytes: __(30)__ /HPF   ——— Granular
  (Isomorphic)/ Dysmorphic
                           Pathologic:
Leukocytes: __4__ /HPF   ——— Broad
                           ——— Fatty
Micro-organisms: Bacteria   ——— Cellular (RBC, WBC, RTC)
            Fungus   ——— Blood (heme-granular)
            Parasites   ——— Waxy

Epithelial cells: Squamous   *Lipid:*   Noncellular
           Urothelial (Moderate)   Cellular
           Renal

                          Epithelial fragments: (Several)

                          Epithelial abnormalities:

INTERPRETATION:
Isomorphic hematuria, epithelial
fragment consistent with
instrumentation.

Comment: ——————————————
——————————————————
——————————————————

RECOMMENDATIONS:
____ Microbiologic studies
____ Renal function test
____ Cytodiagnostic urinalysis
____ Other: _____

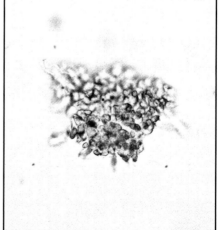

Wet Urinalysis

HEMATURIA—NEOPLASIA

AGE ___40___

SEX ___M___

SPECIMEN TYPE ___Random void___

CLINICAL INFORMATION: Asymptomatic microhematuria.

MACROSCOPIC DESCRIPTION:

Color: ___Yellow___ *Clarity:* ___Clear___   *Specific Gravity:* ___1.015___ *Volume:* ___20___ ml

---

URINE CHEMISTRY:

Reagent Strip:

   pH ___5___   Blood (1+)   Protein _NEG_   Glucose ___NEG___   Ketones _NEG_
   Leukocytes (Trace) Nitrite _NEG_   Bilirubin _NEG_   Urobilinogen _NEG_

Confirmatory Studies: SSA ___< 5 mg/dL___   Ictotest _____   Clinitest _____

MICROSCOPIC EVALUATION:

Background:
    Crystals:
    Other (specify):

Erythrocytes: (20) /HPF
   (Isomorphic)/ Dysmorphic

Leukocytes: ___3___ /HPF

Micro-organisms: Bacteria
                Fungus
                Parasites

Epithelial cells: Squamous
                Urothelial (Moderate)
                Renal

Casts: _____ /LPF:

Physiologic:
    —— Hyaline
    —— Granular

Pathologic:
    —— Broad
    —— Fatty
    —— Cellular (RBC, WBC, RTC)
    —— Blood (heme-granular)
    —— Waxy

Lipid: Noncellular
          Cellular

Epithelial fragments:

Epithelial abnormalities: (Suspect urothelial)

INTERPRETATION:

Isomorphic hematuria. Urothelial
abnormality present.

Comment: ——————————————

RECOMMENDATIONS:

_____ Microbiologic studies
_x_ Cytodiagnostic urinalysis
_____ Renal function test
_____ Other: _____

HEMATURIA—RENAL DISORDER

AGE __N/A__

SEX __N/A__   **SPECIMEN TYPE** ___Random void___

CLINICAL INFORMATION: Post-streptococcal infection, hematuria.

MACROSCOPIC DESCRIPTION:
Color: (**Brown**)   *Clarity:* (**Cloudy**)   *Specific Gravity:* __1.015__   *Volume:* __20__ mL

URINE CHEMISTRY:
Reagent Strip:
    pH __5__   Blood (**3+**)   Protein (**3+ (500mg/dL)**) Glucose __NEG__   Ketones __NEG__
    Leukocytes (**1+**)   Nitrite __NEG__   Bilirubin __NEG__   Urobilinogen __NEG__

Confirmatory Studies: SSA (**500 mg/dL**)   Ictotest _____   Clinitest _____

MICROSCOPIC EVALUATION:

Background: (**Dirty**)
    Crystals :
    Other (specify):

Erythrocytes: (**25**) /HPF
(**Isomorphic / Dysmorphic**)

Leukocytes: (**8**) /HPF

Micro-organisms: Bacteria
               Fungus
               Parasites

Epithelial cells: Squamous
               Urothelial (- **Few**)
               Renal

Casts: (**2-4**) /LPF:

Physiologic:
    __0-1__ Hyaline
    __0-1__ Granular

Pathologic:
    _____ Broad
    _____ Fatty
    (**0-1**) Cellular (**RBC** WBC, RTC)
    (**3**) (**Blood (heme-granular)**)
    _____ Waxy

Lipid: Noncellular
         Cellular

Epithelial fragments:

Epithelial abnormalities:

INTERPRETATION:
 __Renal bleeding, pathologic casts__
 __and proteinuria present. Suspect__
 __glomerular bleeding/damage.__

Comment: _____

_____

_____

RECOMMENDATIONS:
_____ Microbiologic studies
__X__ Cytodiagnostic urinalysis
_____ Renal function test
_____ Other: _____

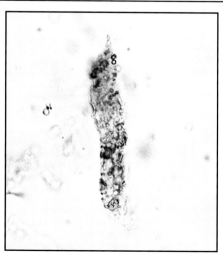

Figure 3. Algorithm and Correlations for Dipstick Leukocyte Esterasuria

---

CLINICAL CONDITIONS:

	Physiologic		Pathologic			
	(Stress, Exercise)	Infection	Inflammation	Lithiasis	Neoplasia	Renal Disorder

---

Case Correlative

Examples:		Case #6	Case #7			Case #8

URINALYSIS FINDINGS:

Physical
    Color   ←———————————— Yellow ————————————→
    Appearance   ←———————— 1 – 4+ Turbidity ————————→

Chemistry
    Leukocyte Esterase   ←——————— 1 – 4+ ———————→
    Nitrite   ←Positive———→

Cells
    RBCs   ←————— Iso/Dys RBCs ————————→
    WBCs   ←————— 1 – 4+ WBCs ————————→
    RTCs

Casts   Pathologic (WBC)

Crystals   Occasional

Concretions   Present

Microbiology   >2+ Bacteria
                           >2+ Fungi
                           Parasites

Epithelial Abnormalities   Abnormal cells and/or fragments
                                       Suspect renal fragment

---

dys=dysmorphic   iso=isomorphic   occ=occasional   RTC=renal tubular cell

---

AGE __50__
SEX __M__   **SPECIMEN TYPE** __First morning void__

CLINICAL INFORMATION: Painful urination.

MACROSCOPIC DESCRIPTION:
Color: __Yellow__   Clarity: (Cloudy)   Specific Gravity: __1.015__   Volume: __50__ mL

URINE CHEMISTRY:
Reagent Strip:
    pH __6__   Blood (Trace)   Protein __NEG__   Glucose __NEG__   Ketones __NEG__
    Leukocytes (POS)   Nitrite (POS)   Bilirubin __NEG__   Urobilinogen __NEG__

Confirmatory Studies: SSA __< 5 mg/dL__   IctoTest _____   CliniTest _____

MICROSCOPIC EVALUATION:
Background: (Dirty)   Casts: _____ /LPF:
    Crystals :
    Other (specify): Mucus   Physiologic:
                    —— Hyaline
Erythrocytes: __2__ /HPF   —— Granular
    (Isomorphic)/ Dysmorphic
                        Pathologic:
Leukocytes: (>50) /HPF   —— Broad
                        —— Fatty
Micro-organisms: Bacteria (3+)   —— Cellular (RBC, WBC, RTC)
               Fungus   —— Blood (heme-granular)
               Parasites   —— Waxy

Epithelial cells: Squamous __Few__
               Urothelial (Many)   Lipid: Noncellular
               Renal   Cellular

                                        Epithelial fragments:

                                        Epithelial abnormalities:

INTERPRETATION:
__Leukocyturia and bacteriuria present.__
__Suspect bacterial UTI.__

Comment:_____

RECOMMENDATIONS:
__X__ Microbiologic studies
_____ Cytodiagnostic urinalysis
_____ Renal function test
_____ Other:

Wet Urinalysis

LEUKOCYTURIA—INFLAMMATION

AGE __25__
SEX __F__

SPECIMEN TYPE __First-morning void__

CLINICAL INFORMATION: Dysuria, frequency.

MACROSCOPIC DESCRIPTION:
Color: __Yellow__ *Appearance:* __Cloudy__ *Specific Gravity:* __1.015__ *Volume:* __100__ mL

URINE CHEMISTRY:
Reagent Strip:

pH __6__	Blood (**Trace**)	Protein __NEG__	Glucose __NEG__	Ketones __NEG__
Leukocytes (**POS**)	Nitrite __NEG__	Bilirubin __NEG__	Urobilinogen __NEG__	

Confirmatory Studies: SSA __< 5 mg/dL__

MICROSCOPIC EVALUATION:
Background: Slightly Dirty
    Crystals :
    Other (specify): Mucus

Erythrocytes: __1__ /HPF
    Isomorphic / Dysmorphic

Leukocytes: (__10__) /HPF

Micro-organisms: Bacteria
                Fungus
                Parasites

Epithelial cells: Squamous - Few
                Urothelial - Few
                Renal

Casts: __0__ /LPF:

Physiologic:
    ——— Hyaline
    ——— Granular

Pathologic:
    ——— Broad
    ——— Fatty
    ——— Cellular (RBC, WBC, RTC)
    ——— Blood (heme-granular)
    ——— Waxy

Lipid: Noncellular
           Cellular

Epithelial fragments:

Epithelial abnormalities:

INTERPRETATION:
Leukocyturia.

Comment: ————————————

RECOMMENDATIONS:
_____ Microbiologic studies
_____ Cytodiagnostic urinalysis
_____ Renal function test
_____ Other:

AGE   N/A

SEX   N/A   **SPECIMEN TYPE**   Random void

CLINICAL INFORMATION: Prior urinary tract infection (UTI).

MACROSCOPIC DESCRIPTION:
Color: Yellow   *Clarity:* Slighty Cloudy   *Specific Gravity:* 1.015   *Volume:*   50 mL

URINE CHEMISTRY:
Reagent Strip:
    pH   6   Blood (1+)   Protein NEG   Glucose NEG   Ketones NEG
    Leukocytes (POS) Nitrite (POS)   Bilirubin NEG   Urobilinogen NEG

Confirmatory Studies: SSA   < 5 mg/dL   IctoTest _____   CliniTest _____

MICROSCOPIC EVALUATION:

Background: Slightly Dirty
    Crystals :
    Other (specify): Mucus

Erythrocytes: (5) /HPF
    (Isomorphic)/ Dysmorphic

Leukocytes: (25) /HPF

Micro-organisms: Bacteria
                Fungus
                Parasites

Epithelial cells: Squamous
                Urothelial   Few
                Renal

Casts: 0-1 /LPF:

    Physiologic:
        —— Hyaline
        —— Granular

    Pathologic:
        —— Broad
        —— Fatty
      (1) —— Cellular (RBC (WBC) RTC)
        —— Blood (heme-granular)
        —— Waxy

Lipid: Noncellular
        Cellular

Epithelial fragments:

Epithelial abnormalities:

INTERPRETATION:
Isomorphic hematuria and leukocyturia. Cellular
pathologic cast noted. Suspect tubulointerstitial
inflammation (possible ascending infection).

Comment: _____

RECOMMENDATIONS:
_____ Microbiologic studies
__x__ Cytodiagnostic urinalysis
_____ Renal function test
_____ Other:

Figure 4. Algorithm and Correlations for Proteinuria

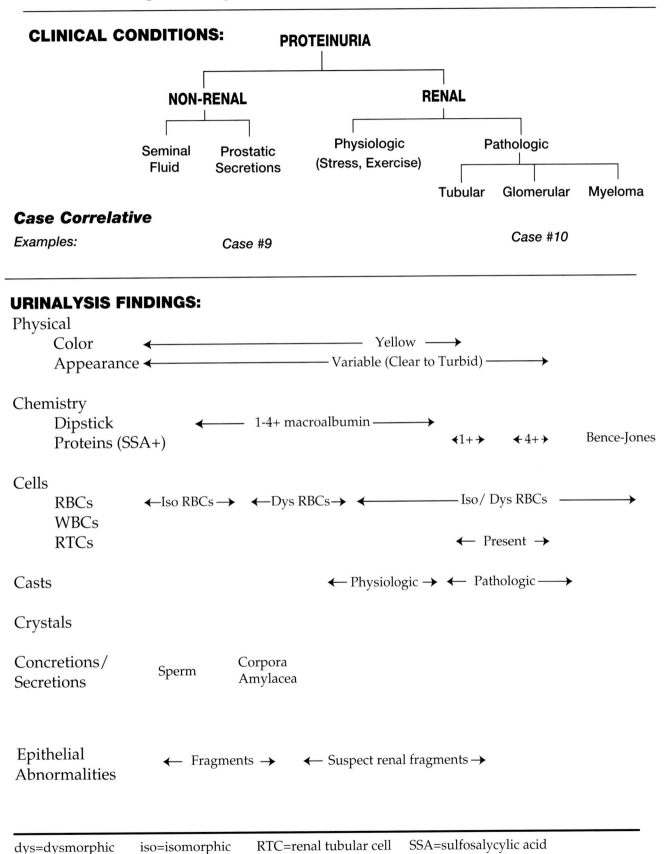

CLINICAL CONDITIONS:

PROTEINURIA
- NON-RENAL
  - Seminal Fluid
  - Prostatic Secretions
- RENAL
  - Physiologic (Stress, Exercise)
  - Pathologic
    - Tubular
    - Glomerular
    - Myeloma

Case Correlative

Examples: Case #9   Case #10

URINALYSIS FINDINGS:

Physical
    Color   ←———————————— Yellow ————→
    Appearance ←——————— Variable (Clear to Turbid) ————→

Chemistry
    Dipstick   ←——— 1-4+ macroalbumin ———→
    Proteins (SSA+)   ←1+→   ←4+→   Bence-Jones

Cells
    RBCs ←Iso RBCs→ ←Dys RBCs→ ←——— Iso/Dys RBCs ————→
    WBCs
    RTCs   ←— Present →

Casts   ←— Physiologic → ←— Pathologic ———→

Crystals

Concretions/   Sperm   Corpora
Secretions   Amylacea

Epithelial   ←— Fragments → ←— Suspect renal fragments →
Abnormalities

dys=dysmorphic   iso=isomorphic   RTC=renal tubular cell   SSA=sulfosalycylic acid

PROTEINURIA—PROSTATIC SECRETIONS

AGE 65
SEX M

SPECIMEN TYPE Random void

CLINICAL INFORMATION: Dysuria and frequency.

MACROSCOPIC DESCRIPTION:
Color: Dark Yellow Clarity: Slightly Cloudy *Specific Gravity:* 1.010 *Volume:* 15 mL

URINE CHEMISTRY:
Reagent Strip:
   pH 6 Blood 1+ Protein Trace (15 mg/dL) Glucose NEG Ketones NEG
   Leukocytes 1+ Nitrite NEG Bilirubin NEG Urobilinogen NEG

Confirmatory Studies: SSA 10 mg/dL Ictotest _____ Clinitest _____

MICROSCOPIC EVALUATION:
Background: Slightly Dirty
   Crystals:
   Other (specify): Corpora Amylacea
                    Globules
Erythrocytes: 12 /HPF
   Isomorphic / Dysmorphic

Leukocytes: 20 /HPF

Micro-organisms: Bacteria
                    Fungus
                    Parasites

Epithelial cells: Squamous
                     Urothelial
                     Renal

Casts: _____ /LPF:

   Physiologic:
   —— Hyaline
   —— Granular

   Pathologic:
   —— Broad
   —— Fatty
   —— Cellular (RBC, WBC, RTC)
   —— Blood (heme-granular)
   —— Waxy

Lipid: Noncellular
          Cellular

Epithelial fragments:

Epithelial abnormalities:

INTERPRETATION:
<u>Isomorphic hematuria and leukocyturia. Corpora amylacea indicating prostatic secretions. Globules present indicating obstructive uropathy.</u>

Comment: _____
_____
_____

RECOMMENDATIONS:
_____ Microbiologic studies
_____ Cytodiagnostic urinalysis

Wet Urinalysis

PROTEINURIA—GLOMERULAR

AGE __50__
SEX __M__   SPECIMEN TYPE __Random void__

CLINICAL INFORMATION: Renal failure, hematuria.

MACROSCOPIC DESCRIPTION:
Color: __Yellow__   *Appearance:* __Cloudy__   *Specific Gravity:* __1.010__   *Volume:* __20__ ml

URINE CHEMISTRY:
Reagent Strip:
    pH __7__   Blood (1+)   Protein (3+ (500 mg/dL))   Glucose __NEG__   Ketones __NEG__
    Leukocytes (1+)   Nitrite __NEG__   Bilirubin __NEG__   Urobilinogen __NEG__

Confirmatory Studies: SSA (500 mg/dL)

MICROSCOPIC EVALUATION:
Background: Dirty, proteinaceous debris
    Crystals:
    Other (specify):

Erythrocytes: __10__ /HPF
    (Isomorphic)/(Dysmorphic)

Leukocytes: __6__ /HPF

Micro-organisms: Bacteria (Trace)
               Fungus
               Parasites

Epithelial cells: Squamous
               Urothelial (Few)
               Renal (Few)

Casts: (4 - 6) /LPF:

  Physiologic:
    __2__ Hyaline
    __2__ Granular

  Pathologic:
    _____ Broad
    (0-1 **Fatty**)
    _____ Cellular (RBC, WBC, RTC)
    _____ Blood (heme-granular)
    (__2__ **Waxy**)

Lipid: Noncellular
          Cellular (**Renal Cells (Lipid-Laden)**)

Epithelial fragments: (**Suspect Renal**)

Epithelial abnormalities:

INTERPRETATION:
Isomorphic/dysmorphic hematuria. Proteinuria
pathologic casts and possible renal fragments.
Fatty cast and lipid-laden renal cells consistent
with nephrotic syndrome.

Comment: —————————————

RECOMMENDATIONS:
_____ Microbiologic studies
__x__ Cytodiagnostic urinalysis
__x__ Renal function test
_____ Other:

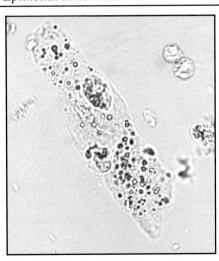

Figure 5. Algorithm and Correlations for Glucosuria

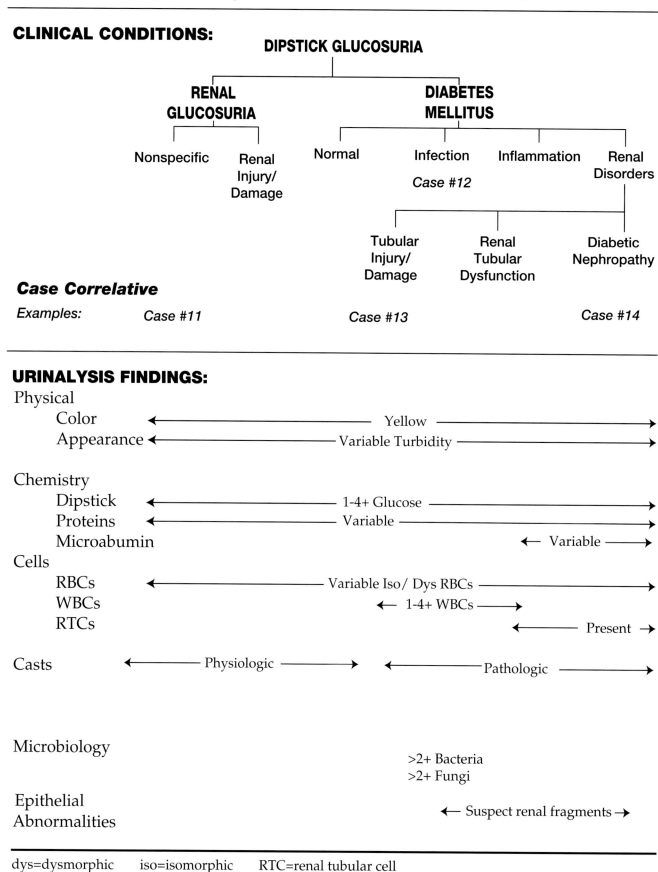

CLINICAL CONDITIONS:

DIPSTICK GLUCOSURIA

RENAL GLUCOSURIA

Nonspecific   Renal Injury/ Damage

DIABETES MELLITUS

Normal   Infection   Inflammation   Renal Disorders

Case #12

Tubular Injury/ Damage   Renal Tubular Dysfunction   Diabetic Nephropathy

Case Correlative

Examples: *Case #11*   *Case #13*   *Case #14*

URINALYSIS FINDINGS:

Physical
 Color ←——————— Yellow ———————→
 Appearance ←——————— Variable Turbidity ———————→

Chemistry
 Dipstick ←——————— 1-4+ Glucose ———————→
 Proteins ←——————— Variable ———————→
 Microabumin ←— Variable —→

Cells
 RBCs ←——————— Variable Iso/ Dys RBCs ———————→
 WBCs ←— 1-4+ WBCs —→
 RTCs ←——— Present →

Casts ←——— Physiologic ———→   ←——— Pathologic ———→

Microbiology
 >2+ Bacteria
 >2+ Fungi

Epithelial Abnormalities ←— Suspect renal fragments →

dys=dysmorphic   iso=isomorphic   RTC=renal tubular cell

Wet Urinalysis

96

CASE #11

GLUCOSURIA—RENAL GLUCOSURIA, NONSPECIFIC

AGE __40__
SEX __N/A__

SPECIMEN TYPE __Random void__

CLINICAL INFORMATION: Annual physical exam.

MACROSCOPIC DESCRIPTION:
Color: __Yellow__ *Appearance:* __Cloudy__ *Specific Gravity:* __1.015__ *Volume:* __60__ mL

URINE CHEMISTRY:
Reagent Strip:
  pH __6__ Blood __NEG__ Protein __NEG__ Glucose ⟨2+ (100 mg/dL)⟩ Ketones __NEG__
  Leukocytes __NEG__ Nitrite __NEG__ Bilirubin __NEG__ Urobilinogen __NEG__

Confirmatory Studies: SSA __< 5 mg/dL__

MICROSCOPIC EVALUATION:

Background: Clean
   Crystals :
   Other (specify):

Erythrocytes: __2__ /HPF
   ⟨Isomorphic⟩/ Dysmorphic

Leukocytes: __0__ /HPF

Micro-organisms: Bacteria
          Fungus
          Parasites

Epithelial cells: Squamous - Rare
           Urothelial
           Renal

Casts: __0 - 1__ /LPF:

Physiologic:
   __0-1__ Hyaline
   ―――― Granular

Pathologic:
   ―――― Broad
   ―――― Fatty
   ―――― Cellular (RBC, WBC, RTC)
   ―――― Blood (heme-granular)
   ―――― Waxy

Lipid: Noncellular
       Cellular

Epithelial fragments:

Epithelial abnormalities:

INTERPRETATION:
Glucosuria present. Suspect renal glucosuria.

Comment: __Diabetes should be excluded.__

RECOMMENDATIONS:
_____ Microbiologic studies
_____ Cytodiagnostic urinalysis
_____ Renal function test
_____ Other:

Appendix 1: Algorithms and Correlations

97

GLUCOSURIA—DIABETES MELLITUS, INFECTION

AGE __30__

SEX __F__

SPECIMEN TYPE ___Random void___

CLINICAL INFORMATION: Dysuria.

MACROSCOPIC DESCRIPTION:
Color: __Yellow__   *Clarity:* __Slighty Cloudy__   *Specific Gravity:* __1.015__   *Volume:* __70__ mL

URINE CHEMISTRY:
Reagent Strip:
   pH ___6___   Blood (**Trace**)   Protein (**15 mg/dL**)   Glucose (**2+ (100 mg/dl)**)   Ketones __NEG__
   Leukocytes (**POS**)   Nitrite (**POS**)   Bilirubin __NEG__   Urobilinogen __NEG__

Confirmatory Studies: SSA __< 5 mg/dL__   IctoTest _____   CliniTest _____

MICROSCOPIC EVALUATION:
Background: (**Dirty**)
   Crystals:
   Other (specify): Mucus

Erythrocytes: __2__ /HPF
   (**Isomorphic**) Dysmorphic

Leukocytes: (**> 50**) /HPF

Micro-organisms: Bacteria
                      Fungus (**Budding Yeast**)
                      Parasites

Epithelial cells: Squamous Few
                       Urothelial Few
                       Renal

Casts: _____ /LPF:

Physiologic:
   —— Hyaline
   —— Granular

Pathologic:
   —— Broad
   —— Fatty
   —— Cellular (RBC, WBC, RTC)
   —— Blood (heme-granular)
   —— Waxy

Lipid: Noncellular
            Cellular

Epithelial fragments:

Epithelial abnormalities:

INTERPRETATION:
<u>Leukocyturia and funguria. Suspect fungal UTI.</u>

Comment: _____

RECOMMENDATIONS:
__x__ Microbiologic studies
_____ Cytodiagnostic urinalysis
_____ Renal function test
_____ Other:

Wet Urinalysis

GLUCOSURIA— TUBULAR INJURY/DAMAGE

AGE __5__
SEX __M__

SPECIMEN TYPE __Random void__

CLINICAL INFORMATION: Oliguric, vomiting, and lethargic.

MACROSCOPIC DESCRIPTION:
Color: Dark Yellow *Clarity:* (Cloudy) *Specific Gravity:* 1.020 *Volume:* __5__ mL

URINE CHEMISTRY:
Reagent Strip:
   pH __5__ Blood (1+) Protein Trace (15 mg/dL) Glucose (Trace) Ketones __NEG__
   Leukocytes (1+) Nitrite __NEG__ Bilirubin __NEG__ Urobilinogen __NEG__

Confirmatory Studies: SSA (10 mg/dL) Ictotest _____ Clinitest _____

MICROSCOPIC EVALUATION:
Background: Slightly Dirty
   Crystals: (Calcium Oxalate)
   Other (specify):

Erythrocytes: (8) /HPF
(Isomorphic / Dysmorphic)

Leukocytes: (6) /HPF

Micro-organisms: Bacteria
   Fungus
   Parasites

Epithelial cells: Squamous
   Urothelial
   Renal (Many)

Casts: (0 - 2) /lpf:

Physiologic:
   __2__ Hyaline
   __2__ Granular

Pathologic:
   _____ Broad
   _____ Fatty
   (0-1) Cellular (RBC, WBC, (RTC))
   _____ Blood (heme-granular)
   (0-1) (Waxy)

Lipid: Noncellular
   Cellular

Epithelial fragments: (Suspect renal)

Epithelial abnormalities:

INTERPRETATION:
Isomorphic/dysmorphic hematuria.
Leukocyturia. Calcium oxalate crystalluria.
Proteinuria. Pathologic casts and possible renal
cells indicating renal injury.

Comment: _____

RECOMMENDATIONS:
_____ Microbiologic studies
__x__ Cytodiagnostic urinalysis
__x__ Renal function test
_____ Other:

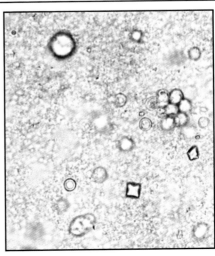

AGE __40__

SEX __F__   SPECIMEN TYPE __Random void__

CLINICAL INFORMATION: Family history of diabetes, proteinuria detected on last exam.

MACROSCOPIC DESCRIPTION:
Color: __Yellow__   *Clarity:* __Clear__   *Specific Gravity:* __1.015__   *Volume:* __60__ mL

URINE CHEMISTRY:
Reagent Strip:

     pH __6__   Blood (**Trace**)   Protein (**100 mg/dL**) Glucose (**3+ (250 mg/dL)**)   Ketones (**1+**)
     Leukocytes (**Trace**) Nitrite __NEG__   Bilirubin __NEG__   Urobilinogen __NEG__

Confirmatory Studies: SSA (**100 mg/dL**)   IctoTest _____   Clinitest _____

MICROSCOPIC EVALUATION:

Background: Slightly Dirty   *Casts:*   (**2-4**) /LPF:
     Crystals :
     Other (specify):   Physiologic:
                                 __0-2__ Hyaline
Erythrocytes: __6__ /HPF   __0-1__ Granular
    (**Isomorphic / Dysmorphic**)
                              Pathologic:
Leukocytes: __4__ /HPF   (**0-1**) (**Broad**)
                                _____ Fatty
Micro-organisms: Bacteria -   Trace   (**0-1**) Cellular (RBC, WBC (**RTC**))
               Fungus   (**0-1**) (**Blood (heme-granular)**)
               Parasites   (**2**) (**Waxy**)

Epithelial cells: Squamous -   Few   *Lipid:*   Noncellular
               Urothelial -   Few   Cellular
               Renal   (**Few**)
                               Epithelial fragments: (**Few, suspect renal**)

                                 Epithelial abnormalities:

INTERPRETATION:
__Isomorphic/dysmorphic hematuria.__
__Glucosuria, proteinuria, and pathologic__
__casts and possible renal fragments.__

Comment: _____

RECOMMENDATIONS:
_____ Microbiologic studies
__x__ Cytodiagnostic urinalysis
__x__ Renal function test
_____ Other:

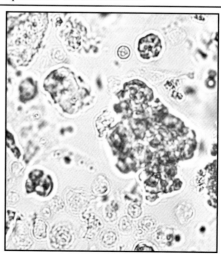

Wet Urinalysis

Plates

Plate 1
Background/Secretions/Concretions

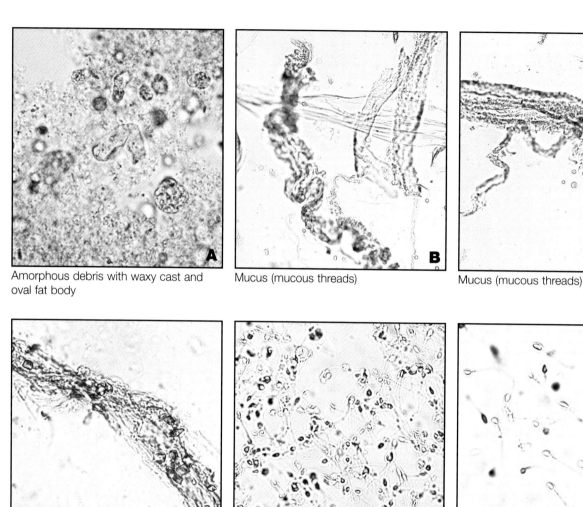

Amorphous debris with waxy cast and oval fat body

Mucus (mucous threads)

Mucus (mucous threads)

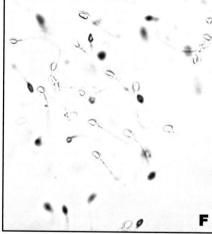

Fibrin

Seminal fluid with spermatozoa

Spermatozoa

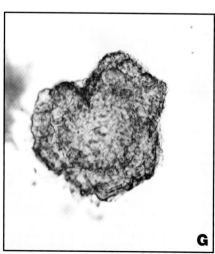

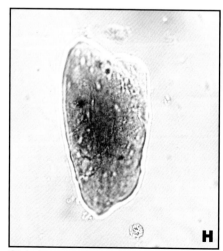

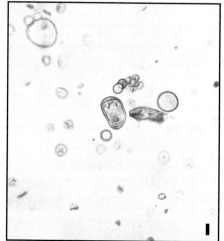

Concretion (microurolithiasis)

Globules

Globules and corpora amylacea

Plate 2
Isomorphic Hematuria/Non-Renal Bleeding
Isomorphic Erythrocytes (RBCs)

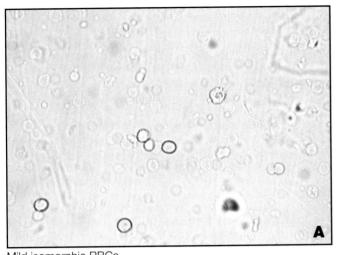

Mild isomorphic RBCs

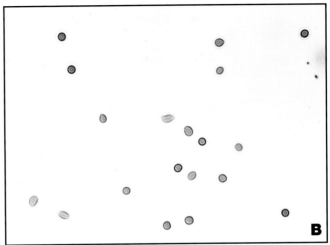

Moderate isomorphic RBCs

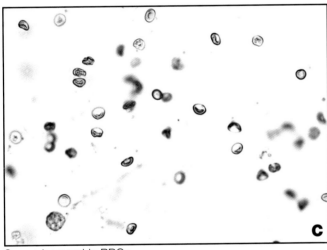

Severe isomorphic RBCs

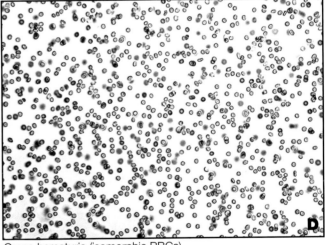

Gross hematuria (isomorphic RBCs)

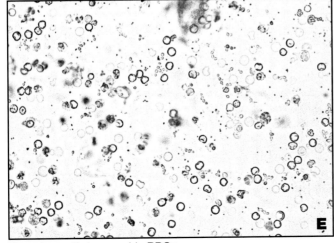

Hypochromatic isomorphic RBCs

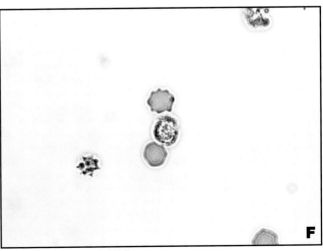

Crenated RBCs and WBC

Appendix 2: Plates

Plate 3

Renal Hematuria/Renal Bleeding
Dysmorphic Erythrocytes (RBCs) and Heme-granular Blood Casts

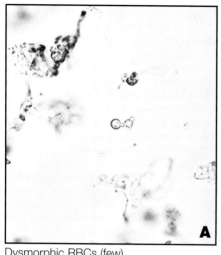

Dysmorphic RBCs (few)

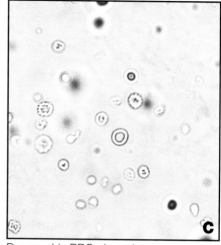

Dysmorphic RBCs (moderate)

Dysmorphic RBCs (many)

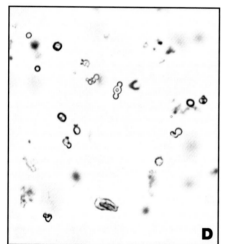

Dysmorphic RBCs (acanthocyte)

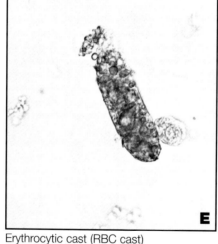

Erythrocytic cast (RBC cast)

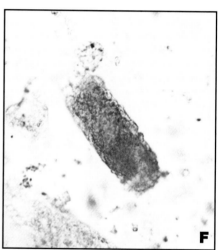

Heme-granular cast (blood cast)

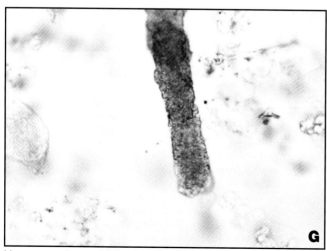

Heme-granular cast (blood cast)

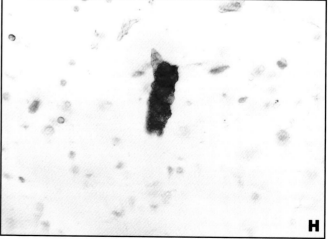

Heme-granular cast (blood cast)

Plate 4

Leukocyturia/Inflammation
Leukocytes (WBCs), Clumps, and Casts

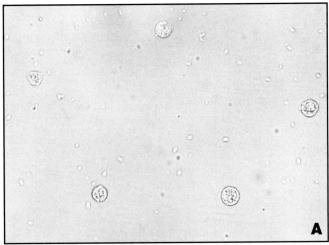

Leukocytes (WBCs) and Bacteria (few)

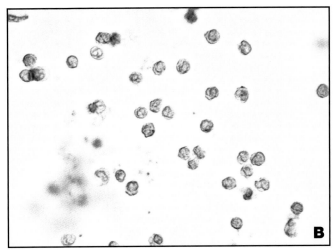

Many WBCs (inflammation)

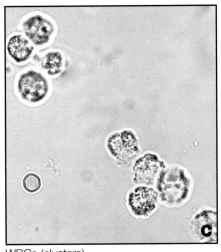

WBCs (clusters)

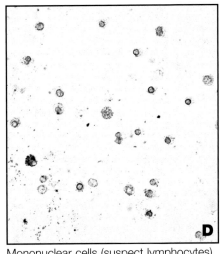

Mononuclear cells (suspect lymphocytes)

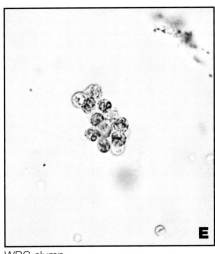

WBC clump

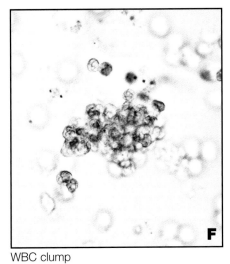

WBC clump

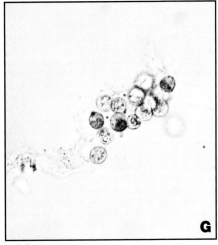

WBC clump

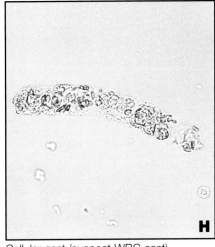

Cellular cast (suspect WBC cast)

Appendix 2: Plates

Plate 5
Bacteriuria
Bacterial Urinary Tract Infection (UTI)

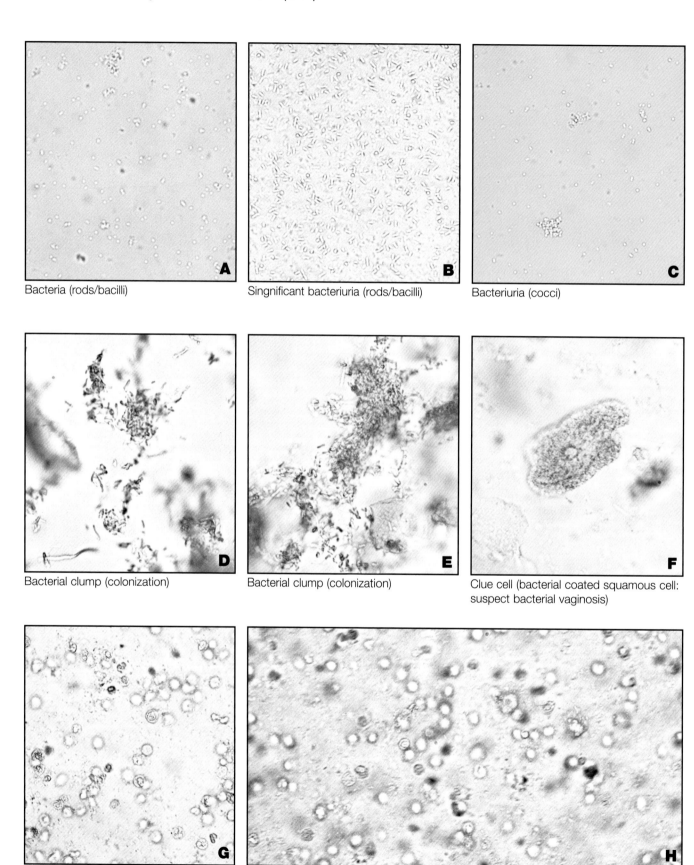

A

Bacteria (rods/bacilli)

B

Singnificant bacteriuria (rods/bacilli)

C

Bacteriuria (cocci)

D

Bacterial clump (colonization)

E

Bacterial clump (colonization)

F

Clue cell (bacterial coated squamous cell:
suspect bacterial vaginosis)

G

Bacterial UTI

H

Bacterial UTI

Plate 6

Funguria/Urinary Parasites
Fungal Urinary Tract Infection (UTI)

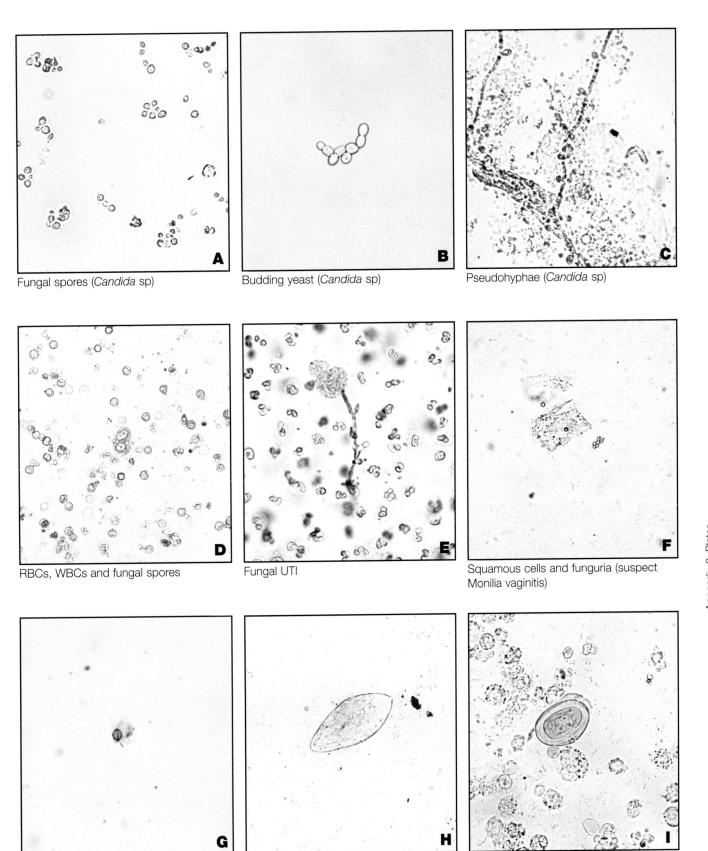

Fungal spores (*Candida* sp)   **A**

Budding yeast (*Candida* sp)   **B**

Pseudohyphae (*Candida* sp)   **C**

RBCs, WBCs and fungal spores   **D**

Fungal UTI   **E**

Squamous cells and funguria (suspect Monilia vaginitis)   **F**

Trichomonad   **G**

Schistosome   **H**

Pinworm   **I**

Appendix 2: Plates

Plate 7
Physiologic Casts

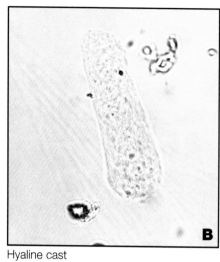

Hyaline cast — A

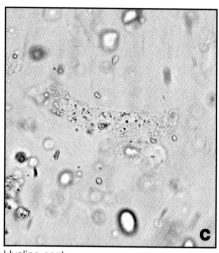

Hyaline cast — C

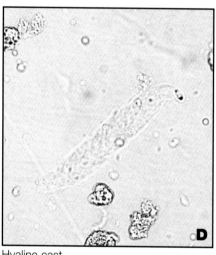

Hyaline cast — D

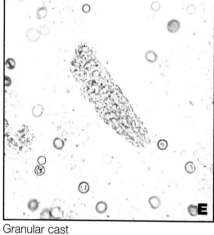

Granular cast — E

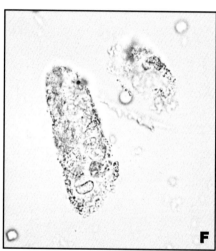

Granular cast — F

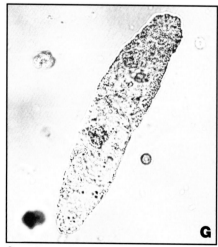

Granular cast — G

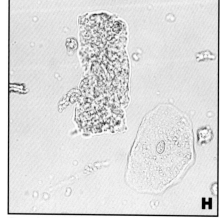

Granular cast — H

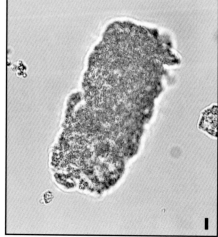

Granular cast — I

Hyaline cast — B

Wet Urinalysis

Plate 8
Pathologic Casts

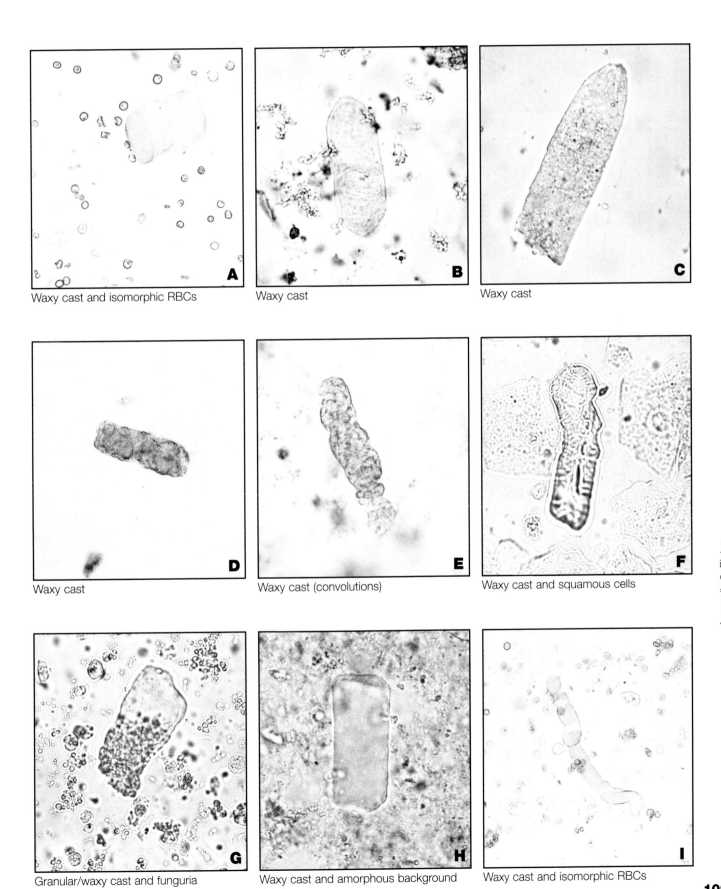

Waxy cast and isomorphic RBCs

Waxy cast

Waxy cast

Waxy cast

Waxy cast (convolutions)

Waxy cast and squamous cells

Granular/waxy cast and funguria

Waxy cast and amorphous background debris

Waxy cast and isomorphic RBCs

Appendix 2: Plates

Plate 8 (continued)
Pathologic Casts

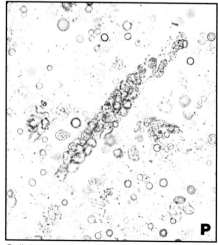

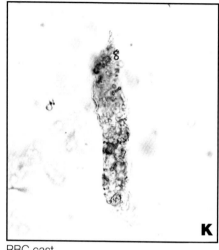

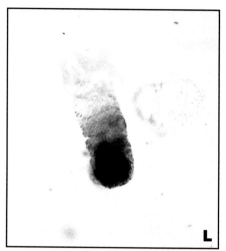

RBC cast

RBC cast

Heme-granular (blood) cast

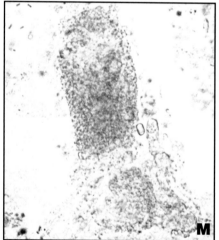

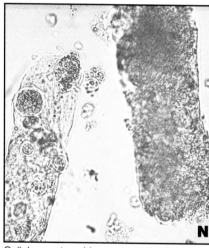

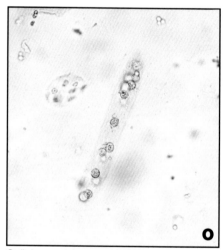

Broad heme-granular (blood) cast

Cellular cast and heme-granular (blood) cast

Cellular cast (suspect WBC cast)

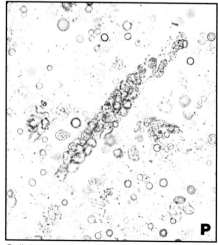

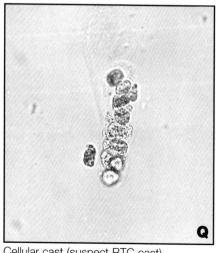

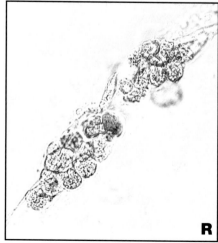

Cellular cast (suspect WBC cast)

Cellular cast (suspect RTC cast)

Cellular cast (suspect RTC cast)

Plate 8 (continued)
Pathologic Casts

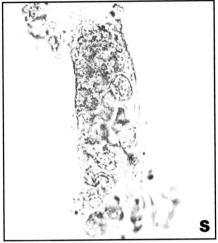

Cellular cast (suspect RTC cast)

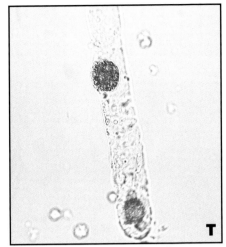

Cellular cast (suspect RTC cast)

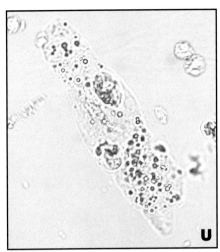

Fatty cast

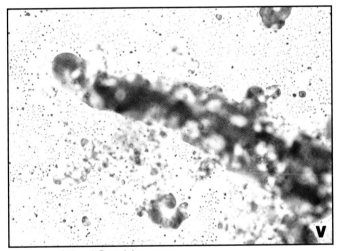

Fatty cast (oil red O stain)

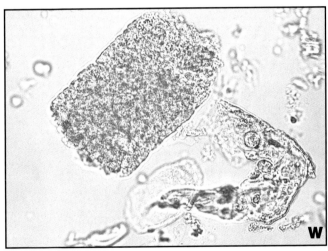

Broad cast

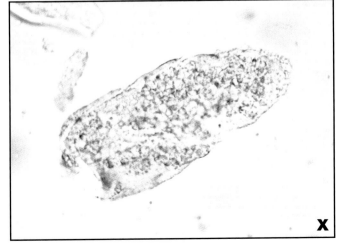

Broad cast

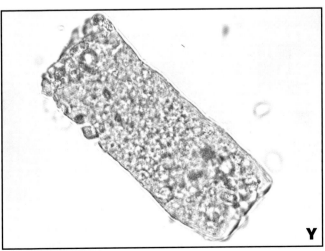

Broad cast

Appendix 2: Plates

111

Plate 9
Normal and Abnormal Squamous Epithelium

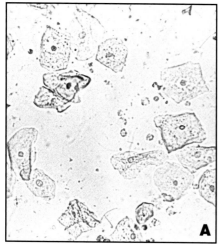

Normal squamous epithelial cells

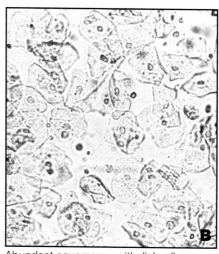

Abundant squamous epithelial cells
(vaginal contamination)

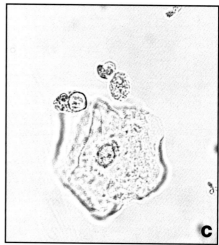

Normal squamous epithelial cell and renal
epithelial cells

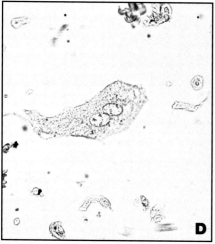

Reactive squamous cells

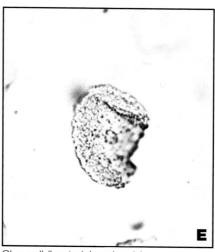

Clue cell (bacterial vaginosis)

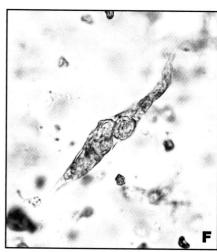

Abnormal squamous cell

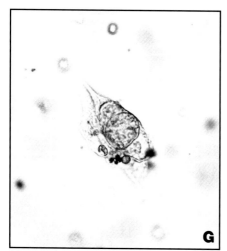

Abnormal squamous cell

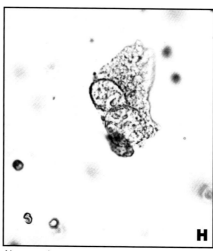

Abnormal squamous cells and isomorphic
RBCs

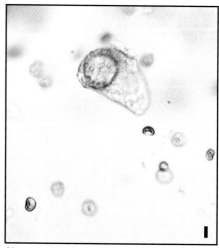

Abnormal squamous cell and isomorphic
RBCs

Plate 10
Normal and Abnormal Urothelium

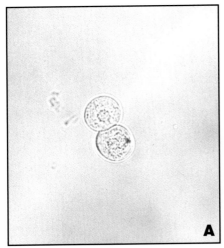

Normal urothelial cells

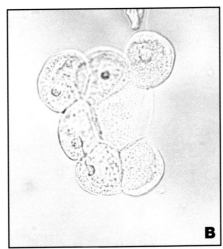

Normal urothelial cells

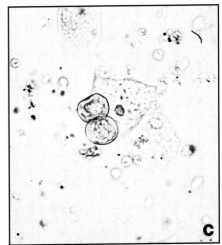

Normal urothelial and squamous cells

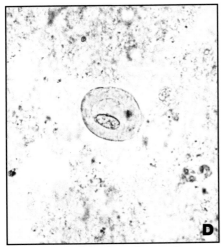

Normal urothelial cells and amorphous debris

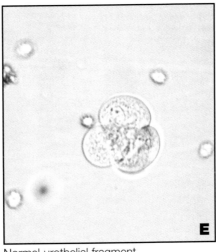

Normal urothelial fragment

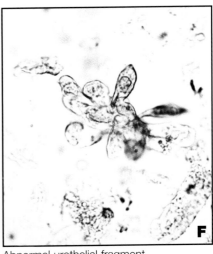

Abnormal urothelial fragment

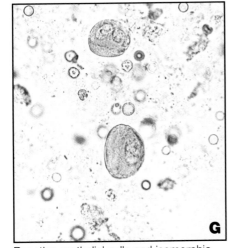

Reactive urothelial cells and isomorphic RBCs

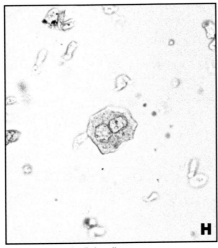

Reactive urothelial cells

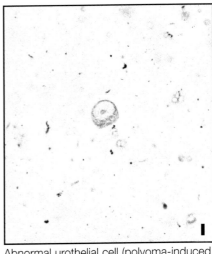

Abnormal urothelial cell (polyoma-induced changes)

Plate 11
Abnormal Urothelium

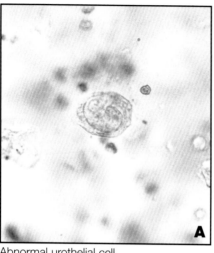

Abnormal urothelial cell

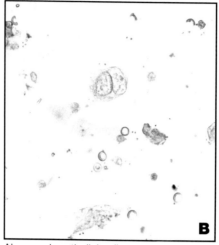

Abnormal urothelial cell

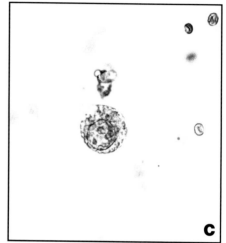

Abnormal urothelial cell

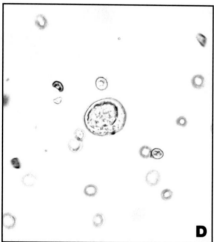

Abnormal urothelial cell and isomorphic RBCs

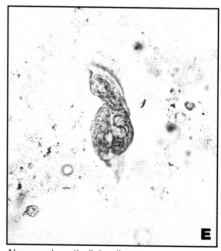

Abnormal urothelial cell

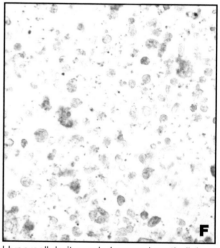

Hypercellularity and abnormal urothelial cells

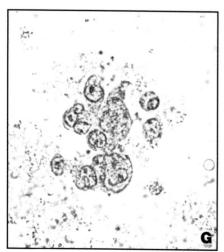

Abnormal urothelial fragment (suspect neoplasia) and amorphous debris

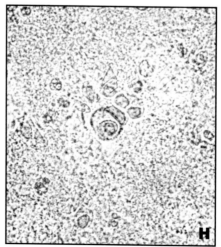

Abnormal urothelial cells (suspect neoplasia) and amorphous debris

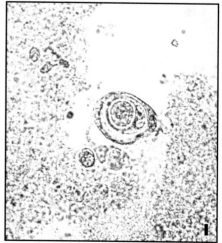

Abnormal urothelial cells (suspect neoplasia) and amorphous debris

Plate 12
Normal and Abnormal Epithelial Fragments

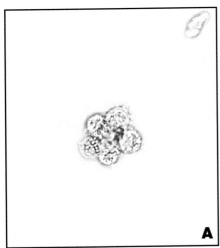

Epithelial fragment

A

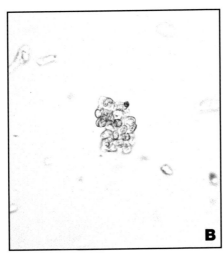

Epithelial fragment

B

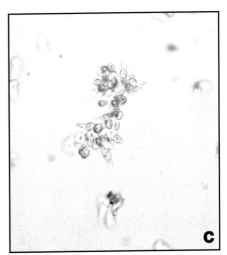

Epithelial fragment

C

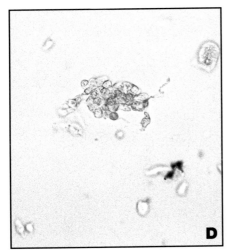

Epithelial fragment (urothelium)

D

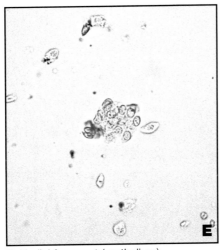

Epithelial fragment (urothelium)

E

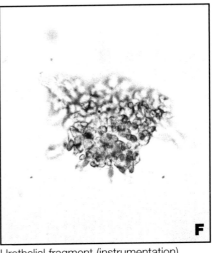

Urothelial fragment (instrumentation)

F

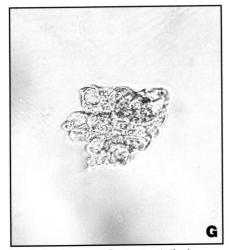

Urothelial fragment (instrumentation)

G

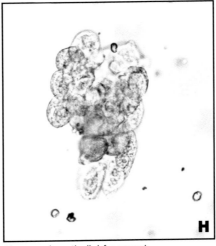

Abnormal urothelial fragment

H

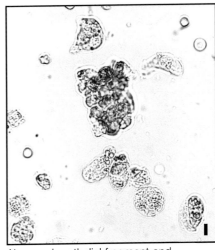

Abnormal urothelial fragment and
isomorphic RBCs (suspect neoplasia)

I

Plate 13
Renal Tubular Injury/Damage

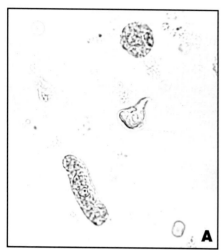

Proximal convoluted renal tubular cells
(RTC)

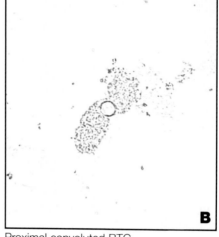

Proximal convoluted RTC

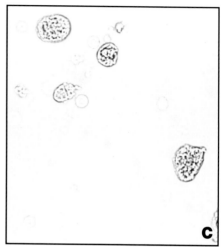

Proximal convoluted RTC

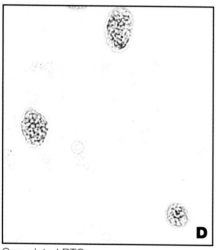

Convoluted RTC

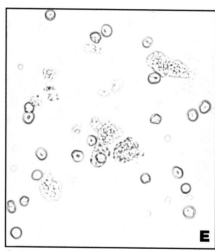

Collecting duct RTC

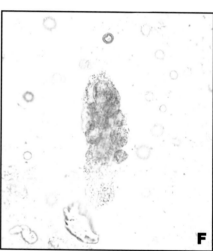

Cellular cast (suspect RTC)

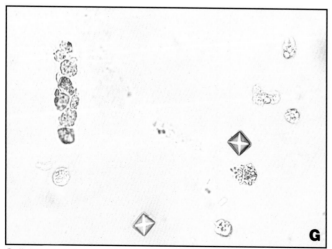

Cellular cast (suspect RTC) and calcium oxalate crystals

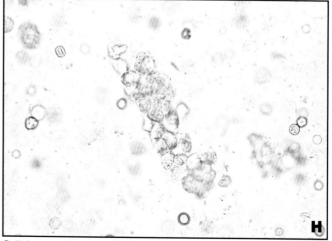

Cellular cast (suspect RTC) and isomorphic RBCs

Plate 13 (continued)
Renal Tubular Injury/Damage

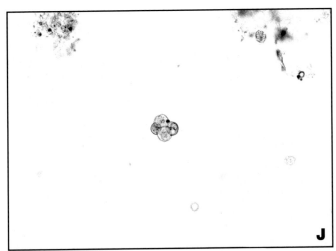

Epithelial fragment (suspect renal fragment)

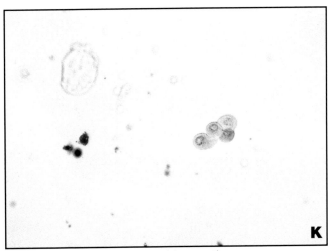

Epithelial fragment (suspect renal fragment)

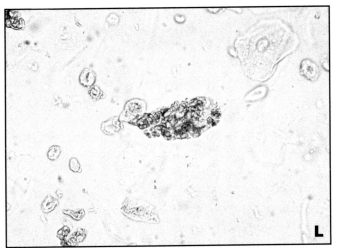

Epithelial fragment (suspect renal fragment)

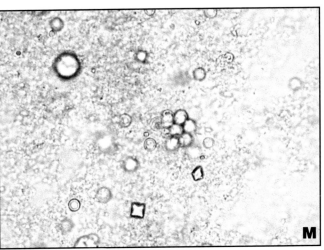

Renal cells and fragment, RBCs, amorphous debris and calcium oxalate crystals

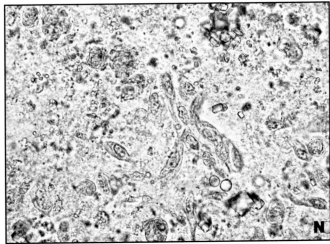

Epithelial fragment and blood cast (suspect chronic renal failure)

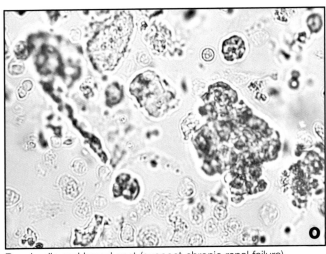

Renal cells and broad cast (suspect chronic renal failure)

Plate 14
Lipiduria/Nephrotic Syndrome

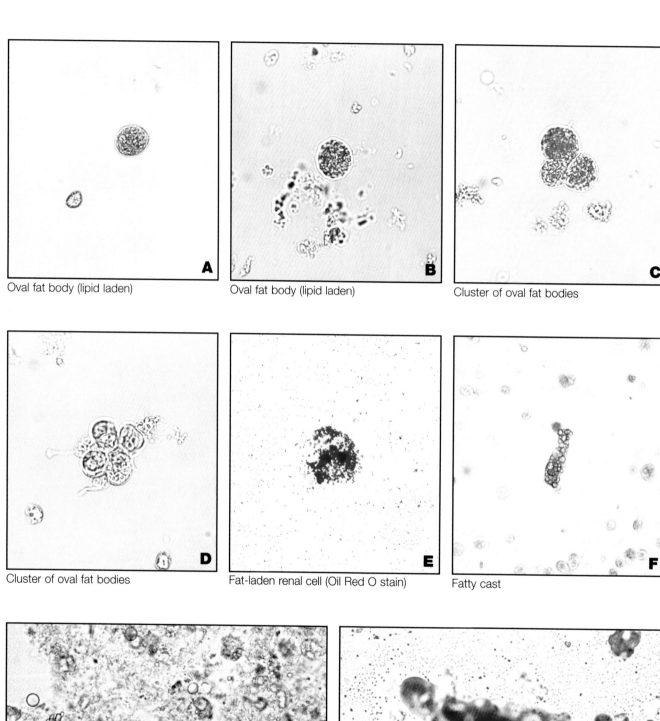

Oval fat body (lipid laden)
A

Oval fat body (lipid laden)
B

Cluster of oval fat bodies
C

Cluster of oval fat bodies
D

Fat-laden renal cell (Oil Red O stain)
E

Fatty cast
F

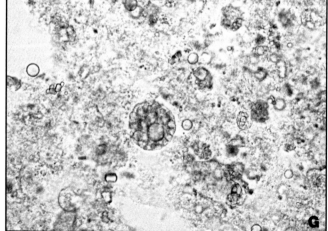

Lipid-laden renal cells, amorphous debris and isomorphic RBCs
G

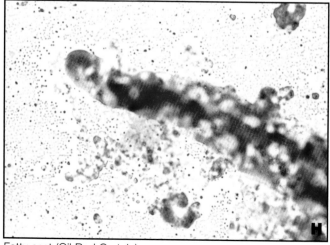

Fatty cast (Oil Red O stain)
H

Wet Urinalysis

Plate 15
Physiologic Crystals

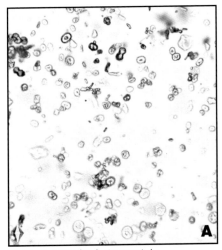

Calcium monohydrate crystals

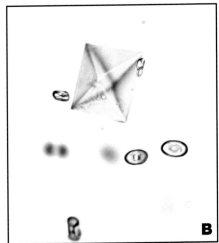

Calcium oxalate crystal (with calcium monohydrate crystals)

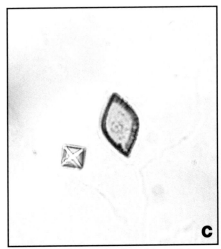

Calcium oxalate and uric acid crystals

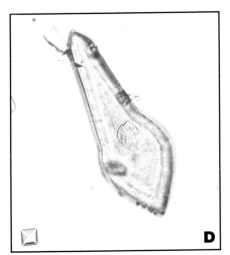

Uric acid crystal

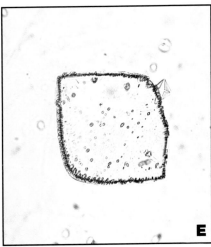

Uric acid crystal

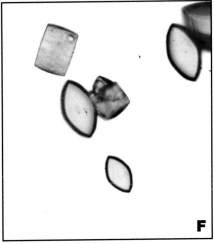

Uric acid crystals

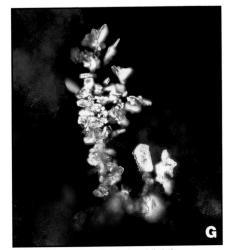

Uric acid crystals (polarized light)

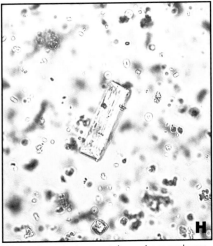

Triple phosphate crystals and amorphous phosphates

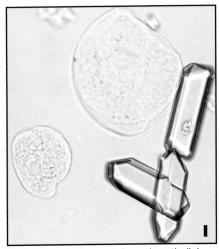

Triple phosphate crystals and urothelial cells

Appendix 2: Plates

119

Plate 16
Pathologic and Drug-Related Crystals

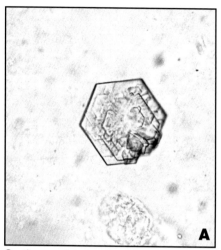

Cystine crystals (cystinuria)

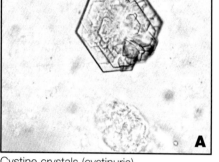

Cystine crystals (cystinuria)

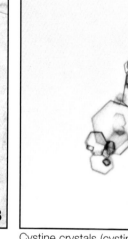

Cystine crystals (cystinuria)

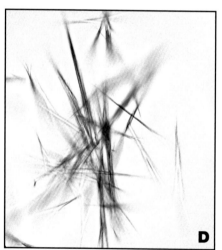

Tyrosine crystals

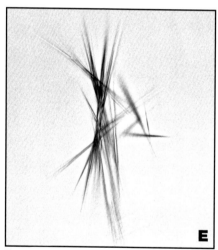

Tyrosine crystals

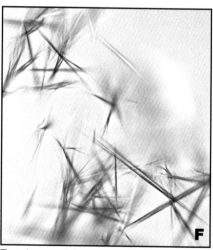

Tyrosine crystals

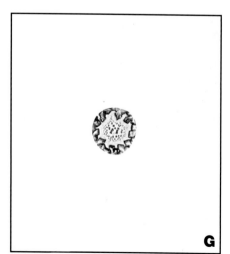

Leucine crystals

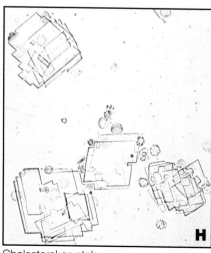

Cholesterol crystals

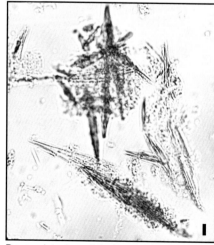

Drug-related crystals (suspect sulfa drugs)

Wet Urinalysis

120

Index

Page numbers in **boldface** indicate figures, tables, and plates.

Wet Urinalysis

Unexplained Epithelial Hypercellularity

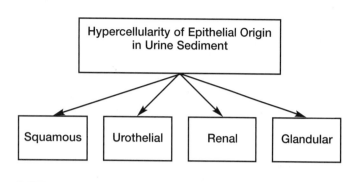

Unexplained Epithelial Fragments of Unknown Origin

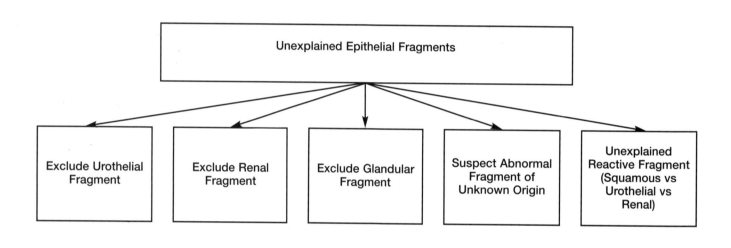

Inflammation of Undetermined Significance

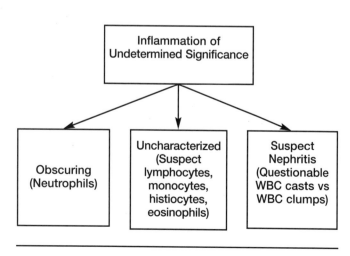